NOURISH

A Cancer-Friendly Cookbook for Healing and Wellness.

Tim Brown

Disclaimer:

This cookbook is intended for informational purposes only and is not a substitute for professional medical advice, diagnosis, or treatment. If the reader requires personal medical or health advice, diagnosis, or treatment, the services of a competent professional should be sought.

INTRODUCTION

Welcome to "Nourish: A Cancer-Friendly Cookbook for Healing and Wellness." In these pages, you'll discover a collection of nutritious recipes, supportive tips, and empowering stories designed to nourish both body and spirit during the journey through cancer.

Living with cancer, whether as a patient, survivor, or caregiver, presents unique challenges. Nutrition plays a vital role in supporting overall health and well-being, helping to manage treatment side effects, boost immunity, and promote healing. However, navigating dietary choices can feel overwhelming amidst the demands of treatment and recovery.

This cookbook aims to simplify the process by providing delicious and nourishing recipes tailored to the needs of those affected by cancer. From energizing breakfasts to comforting main dishes, soothing soups, and satisfying snacks, each recipe is thoughtfully crafted to offer both flavor and nourishment.

But "Nourish" is more than just a collection of recipes. It's a guide to embracing wellness through nourishment, offering practical tips for meal planning, building a cancer-friendly pantry, and practicing mindful eating. It's a source of inspiration and empowerment, featuring stories of resilience and hope from individuals who have walked the cancer journey.

Whether you're seeking ways to support a loved one, looking for nutritious meal ideas during treatment, or simply striving to prioritize your own well-being, "Nourish" is here to accompany you on your path to healing and wellness. Let's embark on this journey together, one nourishing meal at a time.

CHAPTER 1

Understanding Cancer and Nutrition

Nutrition plays a crucial role in cancer prevention, treatment, and overall well-being. In this chapter, we explore the connection between cancer and nutrition, providing insights into how dietary choices can impact health outcomes and quality of life for individuals affected by cancer. Nutrition is a cornerstone of health, and its importance is amplified when facing a cancer diagnosis. In this chapter, we delve deeper into the intricate relationship between cancer and nutrition, exploring how dietary choices can influence the prevention, treatment, and management of cancer.

The Role of Nutrition in Cancer Prevention and Treatment:

We delve into the latest research on how diet and lifestyle factors influence cancer risk and progression. From the importance of consuming a diet rich in fruits, vegetables, whole grains, and lean proteins to the potential benefits of specific nutrients and phytochemicals, we uncover strategies for reducing cancer risk through dietary choices. Mounting evidence suggests that certain dietary patterns and lifestyle factors can impact the development of cancer. We examine the role of nutrition in cancer prevention, highlighting the benefits of a diet rich in antioxidants, fiber, and phytochemicals found in fruits, vegetables, whole grains, and plant-based foods. By adopting a balanced and varied diet, individuals can reduce their risk of developing certain types of cancer and promote overall health and wellness.

Nutrition Strategies during Cancer Treatment:

Cancer treatment can take a toll on the body, leading to a range of side effects that affect appetite, digestion, and nutritional status. From chemotherapy and radiation therapy to surgery and immunotherapy, each treatment modality presents unique challenges and considerations. We explore how nutrition interventions such as dietary modifications, oral nutritional supplements, and hydration strategies can help alleviate treatment-related side effects and support optimal nutrition during therapy.

Addressing Specific Nutritional Needs: Different stages of the

cancer journey may require tailored nutritional approaches to address specific needs and challenges. For example, individuals undergoing chemotherapy may benefit from consuming small, frequent meals to manage nausea and maintain energy levels, while those recovering from surgery may require additional protein and calories to support wound healing and recovery. By understanding these nuances and working closely with healthcare providers and registered dietitians, individuals can optimize their nutrition and enhance their overall well-being.

Navigating Dietary Misconceptions and Myths: The realm

of cancer and nutrition is rife with misinformation and myths. From fad diets promising miracle cures to unsubstantiated claims about superfoods and supplements, it can be challenging to separate fact from fiction. In this section, we debunk common misconceptions and provide evidence-based guidance on making informed dietary choices that are grounded in science and supported by research.

Common Side Effects of Cancer Treatment and How Nutrition Can Help: Cancer treatment can bring about a range of side

effects, including fatigue, nausea, taste changes, and difficulty swallowing. In this section, we discuss how nutrition interventions such as dietary modifications, nutritional supplements, and hydration strategies can help manage these side effects and support overall well-being during treatment.

Tips for Building a Cancer-Friendly Diet: Navigating dietary

choices can be challenging for individuals affected by cancer. Here, we offer practical tips for building a cancer-friendly diet that prioritizes nutrient density, variety, and balance. From incorporating colorful fruits and vegetables to choosing lean proteins and healthy fats, we provide guidance for creating nourishing meals that promote health and healing.

What to eat and avoid

What to Eat

1. **Plant-Based Foods:** Emphasize a diet rich in fruits, vegetables, whole grains, legumes, nuts, and seeds. These foods are packed with vitamins, minerals, antioxidants, and fiber, which play key roles in supporting immune function, reducing inflammation, and promoting overall health.

2. **Lean Proteins:** Incorporate lean sources of protein such as poultry, fish, tofu, legumes, and low-fat dairy into your meals. Protein is essential for tissue repair, immune function, and muscle maintenance, especially during cancer treatment and recovery.

3. **Healthy Fats:** Choose sources of healthy fats such as avocados, nuts, seeds, olive oil, and fatty fish like salmon. These fats provide essential fatty acids and help support heart health and reduce inflammation.

4. **Colorful Fruits and Vegetables:** Aim to include a variety of colorful fruits and vegetables in your diet, as different colors signify different phytonutrients and antioxidants. Fill your plate with a rainbow of produce to ensure you're getting a diverse array of nutrients to support your body's needs.

5. **Whole Grains:** Opt for whole grains such as brown rice, quinoa, oats, barley, and whole wheat bread and pasta. Whole grains provide fiber, vitamins, minerals, and sustained energy, making them a nutritious choice for overall health and well-being.

What Not to Eat:

1. **Processed and Sugary Foods:** Minimize your intake of processed and sugary foods such as sugary beverages, sweets, desserts, and highly processed snacks. These foods offer little nutritional value and can contribute to inflammation, weight gain, and other health issues.

2. **Red and Processed Meats:** Limit consumption of red and processed meats such as beef, pork, bacon, sausage, and deli meats. These meats have been linked to an increased risk of certain cancers and may exacerbate inflammation in the body.

3. **Highly Processed Foods:** Avoid highly processed foods such as fast food, convenience meals, and packaged snacks that are high in unhealthy fats, sodium, and additives. These foods can contribute to poor health outcomes and may increase the risk of chronic diseases.

4. **Excessive Alcohol:** Limit alcohol consumption, as excessive alcohol intake has been linked to an increased risk of certain cancers, including breast, liver, and colorectal cancer. If you choose to drink alcohol, do so in moderation and consider opting for healthier alternatives such as water, herbal tea, or sparkling water with a splash of fruit juice.

By making mindful dietary choices and focusing on nutrient-dense foods, you can support your body's natural healing processes and enhance your overall well-being as you navigate the cancer journey. Remember to consult with your healthcare team or a registered dietitian for personalized nutrition guidance tailored to your individual needs and preferences.

By understanding the intricate relationship between cancer and nutrition, individuals can empower themselves to make informed dietary choices that support their journey through cancer. In this chapter, we lay the foundation for the rest of the book, providing valuable insights and practical tips to help readers harness the power of nutrition for optimal health and well-being.

Also, By gaining a deeper understanding of the intricate interplay between cancer and nutrition, individuals can empower themselves to take an active role in their health and well-being. Armed with knowledge and practical strategies, readers can navigate the complexities of cancer treatment with confidence and resilience, harnessing the power of nutrition to optimize their journey to healing and recovery.

Hydration

Hydration is crucial for individuals affected by cancer, whether they are undergoing treatment or in remission. Here are some key points to consider for cancer-friendly hydration:

1. **Importance of Hydration:** Staying hydrated is essential for overall health and well-being, particularly during cancer treatment. Proper hydration helps maintain fluid balance, supports

digestion, regulates body temperature, and facilitates the transportation of nutrients and oxygen throughout the body.

2. **Increased Fluid Needs:** Cancer treatment, such as chemotherapy and radiation therapy, can increase the risk of dehydration due to side effects such as nausea, vomiting, diarrhea, and loss of appetite. Patients may also experience increased fluid loss through sweating or fever. Therefore, it's important to consume extra fluids to compensate for these losses.

3. **Choosing Hydrating Beverages:** Water is the best choice for hydration, as it is calorie-free and easily accessible. Herbal teas, coconut water, electrolyte drinks, and diluted fruit juices are also good options for maintaining hydration. Avoid sugary drinks and excessive caffeine, as they can contribute to dehydration and may exacerbate certain side effects.

4. **Sipping Throughout the Day:** Encourage individuals to sip fluids consistently throughout the day rather than drinking large amounts at once. This approach can help prevent dehydration and manage treatment-related symptoms such as nausea and vomiting. Using a water bottle or setting reminders can help promote regular hydration.

5. **Monitoring Fluid Intake:** Keep track of fluid intake to ensure adequate hydration, especially during cancer treatment when fluid needs may be higher. Healthcare providers or registered dietitians can provide guidance on recommended daily fluid goals based on individual factors such as age, weight, health status, and treatment regimen.

6. **Addressing Treatment Side Effects:** Certain cancer treatments, such as chemotherapy and radiation therapy, can cause changes in taste perception, dry mouth, and difficulty swallowing, which may affect fluid intake. Encourage patients to experiment with different temperatures, flavors, and textures to find hydrating options that are tolerable and appealing.

7. **Hydration and Nutrition:** Hydration and nutrition are closely intertwined, as many hydrating foods also provide essential nutrients that support overall health and recovery. Fruits, vegetables, soups, and smoothies with high water content can contribute to both hydration and nutritional needs.

8. **Consulting Healthcare Providers:** It's important for individuals affected by cancer to discuss hydration strategies with their healthcare providers or registered dietitians, especially if they

have specific medical conditions or dietary restrictions. Healthcare professionals can offer personalized recommendations and monitor hydration status throughout treatment.

By prioritizing hydration and adopting strategies to maintain fluid balance, individuals affected by cancer can support their overall health and well-being, optimize treatment outcomes, and improve their quality of life during and after cancer treatment.

Meal plan

A cancer-friendly meal plan is designed to provide nourishment and support to individuals undergoing cancer treatment or in remission. It focuses on incorporating nutrient-dense foods that can help boost the immune system, maintain energy levels, and support overall well-being during the challenging journey of battling cancer. Here is a complete 31 days meal plan:

Day	Breakfast	Lunch	Dinner	Snacks	Smoothies
Day 1	Berry Blast Smoothie Bowl	Quinoa Salad	Grilled Salmon with Roasted Vegetables	Carrot Sticks with Hummus	Mixed Berry Smoothie
Day 2	Avocado Breakfast Salad	Lentil Soup with Whole Grain Bread	Vegetable Stir-Fry with Brown Rice	Greek Yogurt with Berries	Green Detox Smoothie
Day 3	Greek Yogurt Parfait	Turkey and Avocado Wrap	Baked Chicken Breast with Quinoa	Almonds	Mango Tango Smoothie
Day 4	Spinach and Feta Egg Muffins	Chickpea Salad	Spaghetti Squash with Marinara Sauce	Apple Slices with Peanut Butter	Blueberry Kale Smoothie
Day 5	Creamy Peanut Butter	Tuna Salad with Quinoa	Grilled Vegetable	Edamame	Pineapple Coconut

Day	Breakfast	Lunch	Dinner	Snacks	Smoothies
	Overnight Oats		Skewers with Quinoa		Smoothie
Day 6	Sweet Potato Breakfast Hash	Chicken Caesar Salad	Lentil Curry with Basmati Rice	Whole Grain Crackers with Cheese	Avocado Banana Smoothie
Day 7	Turmeric Chia Pudding	Hummus and Veggie Plate	Grilled Tofu with Stir-Fried Veggies	Cottage Cheese with Pineapple	Kale Banana Smoothie
Day 8	Banana Walnut Breakfast Cookies	Caprese Salad	Black Bean Tacos with Salsa and Guacamole	Veggie Sticks with Ranch Dip	Strawberry Spinach Smoothie
Day 9	Apple Cinnamon Overnight Oats	Vegetable Soup with Whole Grain Roll	Baked Cod with Roasted Asparagus	Trail Mix	Chocolate Avocado Smoothie
Day 10	Smoked Salmon Breakfast Wrap	Quinoa Stuffed Bell Peppers	Mushroom Risotto	Rice Cakes with Almond Butter	Raspberry Peach Smoothie
Day 11	Pumpkin Pie Chia Pudding	Greek Salad with Grilled Chicken	Spicy Shrimp Stir-Fry with Brown Rice	Yogurt Parfait	Beet Orange Smoothie
Day 12	Green Smoothie	Egg Salad Sandwich	Baked Sweet Potato with Chickpea Salad	Sliced Bell Peppers with Hummus	Tropical Mango Smoothie

Day	Breakfast	Lunch	Dinner	Snacks	Smoothies
Day 13	Almond Butter Banana Toast	Lentil Chili with Cornbread	Grilled Vegetable Pasta Primavera	Kale Chips	Spinach Pineapple Smoothie
Day 14	Tomato and Basil Breakfast Frittata	Spinach and Artichoke Stuffed Chicken	Teriyaki Glazed Salmon with Quinoa	Dark Chocolate Square	Cherry Almond Smoothie
Day 15	Chia Seed Breakfast Pudding	Cobb Salad	Vegetable Curry with Coconut Rice	Greek Yogurt with Granola	Kiwi Blueberry Smoothie
Day 16	Egg and Avocado Toast	Roasted Vegetable Quinoa Bowl	Stuffed Bell Peppers with Cauliflower Rice	Mixed Nuts	Peach Ginger Smoothie
Day 17	Raspberry Coconut Smoothie	Greek Quinoa Salad	Grilled Chicken with Greek Salad	Rice Crackers with Tzatziki	Pomegranate Berry Smoothie
Day 18	Avocado Chocolate Mousse	Mediterranean Veggie Wrap	Baked Turkey Meatballs with Zucchini Noodles	Carrot Sticks with Guacamole	Mango Kiwi Smoothie
Day 19	Spinach and Feta Stuffed Mushrooms	Minestrone Soup with Whole Grain Bread	Blackened Mahi-Mahi with Quinoa	Apple Slices with Almond Butter	Pineapple Spinach Smoothie
Day 20	Frozen Banana Pops	Falafel Salad	Lentil Stew with Whole Grain Roll	Yogurt with Berries	Cherry Vanilla Smoothie

Day	Breakfast	Lunch	Dinner	Snacks	Smoothies
Day 21	Roasted Chickpeas	Antipasto Salad	Veggie Pad Thai with Tofu	Rice Cakes with Peanut Butter	Watermelon Mint Smoothie
Day 22	Spinach and Artichoke Dip	Shrimp and Avocado Salad	Baked Eggplant Parmesan with Whole Wheat Pasta	Celery Sticks with Hummus	Banana Peanut Butter Smoothie
Day 23	Cucumber and Hummus Bites	Mexican Quinoa Salad	Grilled Steak with Sweet Potato Mash	Trail Mix	Oatmeal Cookie Smoothie
Day 24	Berry Yogurt Bark	Asian Slaw with Peanut Dressing	Salmon and Vegetable Foil Packets	Cottage Cheese with Berries	Almond Joy Smoothie
Day 25	Black Bean Hummus	Mediterranean Pasta Salad	Chicken Fajita Bowl with Brown Rice	Whole Grain Crackers with Cheese	Orange Creamsicle Smoothie
Day 26	Carrot Cake Oatmeal	Thai Peanut Zucchini Noodles	Beef Stir-Fry with Quinoa	Veggie Sticks with Hummus	Peanut Butter Banana Smoothie
Day 27	Quinoa-Stuffed Bell Peppers	Kale and Brussels Sprouts Salad	Spaghetti Squash with Turkey Bolognese	Apple Slices with Cheese	Mango Coconut Smoothie
Day 28	Lentil Salad with Lemon Vinaigrette	Grilled Veggie and Goat Cheese Panini	Baked Halibut with Lemon-Dill Sauce	Dark Chocolate Square	Vanilla Berry Smoothie

Day	Breakfast	Lunch	Dinner	Snacks	Smoothies
Day 29	Apple Walnut Quinoa Salad	Southwest Quinoa Bowl	Veggie and Tofu Stir-Fry with Brown Rice	Greek Yogurt with Honey	Strawberry Kiwi Smoothie
Day 30	Greek Yogurt Parfait	Avocado and Tomato Quinoa Bowl	Grilled Pork Tenderloin with Quinoa Salad	Trail Mix	Chocolate Cherry Smoothie
Day 31	Breakfast Burrito	Mediterranean Chickpea Salad	Stuffed Acorn Squash with Wild Rice Pilaf	Rice Cakes with Avocado	Green Tea Smoothie

This meal plan provides a variety of cancer-friendly meals including breakfast, lunch, dinner, snacks, and smoothies for each day of the month.

CHAPTER 2: BREAKFASTS TO START YOUR DAY RIGHT

1. *Berry Blast Smoothie Bowl:*

   - ***Ingredients:*** 1 cup mixed berries (strawberries, blueberries, raspberries), 1 ripe banana, 1 cup spinach, 1/2 cup Greek yogurt, 1/2 cup almond milk, 1/4 cup granola, 2 tablespoons sliced almonds, fresh berries for garnish.

   - ***Instructions:*** In a blender, combine mixed berries, banana, spinach, Greek yogurt, and almond milk. Blend until smooth. Pour into a bowl and top with granola, sliced almonds, and fresh berries.

2. *Creamy Peanut Butter Overnight Oats:*

   - Ingredients: 1/2 cup rolled oats, 1/2 cup almond milk, 2 tablespoons natural peanut butter, 1 tablespoon chia seeds, 1 tablespoon honey or maple syrup.

   - Instructions: In a jar or container, mix rolled oats, almond milk, peanut butter, chia seeds, and honey or maple syrup. Stir well, cover, and refrigerate overnight. Enjoy cold in the morning.

3. *Avocado Breakfast Salad:*

   - ***Ingredients:*** 1 ripe avocado, 1 cup cherry tomatoes, halved, 1/2 cucumber, diced, 2 hard-boiled eggs, sliced, juice of 1/2 lemon, 1 tablespoon olive oil, salt and pepper to taste.

   - ***Instructions:*** In a bowl, combine avocado, cherry tomatoes, cucumber, and hard-boiled eggs. Drizzle with lemon juice and olive oil. Season with salt and pepper to taste.

4. *Quinoa Breakfast Porridge:*

- *Ingredients:* 1/2 cup quinoa, rinsed, 1 cup almond milk, 1/2 teaspoon cinnamon, pinch of salt, 2 tablespoons sliced almonds, 2 tablespoons chopped dates, 1 tablespoon maple syrup.

- *Instructions:* In a saucepan, combine quinoa, almond milk, cinnamon, and salt. Bring to a boil, then reduce heat and simmer for 15-20 minutes, or until quinoa is cooked and liquid is absorbed. Serve topped with sliced almonds, chopped dates, and maple syrup.

5. Sweet Potato Breakfast Hash:

- *Ingredients:* 1 medium sweet potato, diced, 1/2 red bell pepper, diced, 1/4 red onion, diced, 1 cup baby spinach, 1 tablespoon olive oil, salt and pepper to taste, optional: poached egg.

- *Instructions:* In a skillet, heat olive oil over medium heat. Add sweet potato, bell pepper, and onion. Cook until sweet potato is tender and lightly browned, about 10-12 minutes. Add spinach and cook until wilted. Season with salt and pepper. Serve hot, with a poached egg if desired.

6. Greek Yogurt Parfait:

- *Ingredients:* 1/2 cup Greek yogurt, 1/4 cup mixed berries (strawberries, blueberries, raspberries), 2 tablespoons granola, drizzle of honey or maple syrup.

- *Instructions:* In a glass or bowl, layer Greek yogurt, mixed berries, and granola. Repeat layers if desired. Drizzle with honey or maple syrup before serving.

7. Spinach and Feta Egg Muffins:

- *Ingredients:* 4 large eggs, 1 cup baby spinach, chopped, 1/4 cup crumbled feta cheese, 1/4 cup diced red bell pepper, salt and pepper to taste.

- *Instructions:* Preheat oven to 350°F (175°C). In a bowl, whisk together eggs, spinach, feta cheese, bell pepper, salt, and pepper. Pour mixture into greased muffin tins, filling each cup 3/4 full. Bake for 20-25 minutes, or until eggs are set. Allow to cool slightly before serving.

8. Turmeric Chia Pudding:

- *Ingredients*: 1/4 cup chia seeds, 1 cup unsweetened almond milk, 1/2 teaspoon ground turmeric, 1/4 teaspoon ground ginger, 1 tablespoon maple syrup, 1/4 cup diced mango.

- *Instructions:* In a bowl or jar, mix chia seeds, almond milk, turmeric, ginger, and maple syrup. Stir well, cover, and refrigerate for at least 2 hours or overnight, until thickened. Serve topped with diced mango.

9. Smoked Salmon Breakfast Wrap:

- *Ingredients:* 1 whole grain wrap or tortilla, 2 ounces smoked salmon, 1/4 ripe avocado, sliced, 2 tablespoons diced cucumber, 1/4 cup baby arugula, 1 tablespoon cream cheese.

- *Instructions:* Spread cream cheese on the whole grain wrap. Layer smoked salmon, avocado slices, diced cucumber, and baby arugula. Roll up tightly and slice in half before serving.

10. Banana Walnut Breakfast Cookies:

- *Ingredients:* 2 ripe bananas, mashed, 1 cup rolled oats, 1/4 cup chopped walnuts, 1/2 teaspoon ground cinnamon, 1 tablespoon honey or maple syrup.

- *Instructions*: Preheat oven to 350°F (175°C). In a bowl, mix mashed bananas, rolled oats, chopped walnuts, cinnamon, and honey or maple syrup. Drop spoonfuls of the mixture onto a baking sheet lined with parchment paper. Flatten slightly with the back of a spoon. Bake for 15-18 minutes, or until golden brown. Allow to cool before serving.

11. Apple Cinnamon Overnight Oats:

- *Ingredients:*

  - 1/2 cup rolled oats

  - 1/2 cup almond milk

  - 1/2 apple, grated

  - 1 tablespoon maple syrup

  - 1/2 teaspoon cinnamon

- *Instructions:*

1. In a jar or container, mix rolled oats, almond milk, grated apple, maple syrup, and cinnamon. Stir well, cover, and refrigerate overnight. Enjoy cold in the morning.

12. Veggie Breakfast Burrito:

- *Ingredients:*

  - 1 whole grain wrap or tortilla

  - 2 eggs, scrambled

  - 1/4 cup black beans, drained and rinsed

  - 2 tablespoons salsa

  - 1/4 avocado, sliced

  - Fresh cilantro for garnish

- *Instructions:*

1. Fill the whole grain wrap with scrambled eggs, black beans, salsa, and avocado slices.

2. Roll up tightly and garnish with fresh cilantro before serving.

13. Pumpkin Pie Chia Pudding:

- *Ingredients:*

- 1/4 cup chia seeds

- 1 cup coconut milk

- 1/4 cup pumpkin puree

- 1 tablespoon maple syrup

- 1/2 teaspoon pumpkin pie spice

- **Instructions:**

1. In a bowl or jar, mix chia seeds, coconut milk, pumpkin puree, maple syrup, and pumpkin pie spice. Stir well, cover, and refrigerate for at least 2 hours or overnight, until thickened. Serve chilled.

14. Green Smoothie:

- *Ingredients:*

  - 1 cup spinach

  - 1/2 cup kale

  - 1/2 banana

  - 1/2 cup pineapple chunks

  - 1/2 cup coconut water

  - 1 tablespoon chia seeds

- *Instructions:*

1. Blend spinach, kale, banana, pineapple chunks, and coconut water until smooth.

2. Add chia seeds and pulse until combined. Serve immediately.

15. Almond Butter Banana Toast:

- *Ingredients:*

  - 1 slice whole grain bread, toasted

- 1 tablespoon almond butter

- 1/2 banana, sliced

- Drizzle of honey

- *Instructions:*

1. Spread almond butter on the toasted whole grain bread.

2. Top with banana slices and drizzle with honey before serving.

16. Mushroom and Spinach Omelette:

- *Ingredients:*

  - 2 eggs

  - 1/4 cup sliced mushrooms

  - 1/2 cup baby spinach

  - 1 tablespoon grated Parmesan cheese

  - Salt and pepper to taste

- *Instructions:*

1. In a bowl, beat the eggs and season with salt and pepper.

2. Heat a non-stick skillet over medium heat and add sliced mushrooms. Cook until tender.

3. Add baby spinach to the skillet and cook until wilted.

4. Pour the beaten eggs over the mushrooms and spinach. Cook until the edges start to set.

5. Sprinkle grated Parmesan cheese over one half of the omelette. Fold the other half over the cheese and cook until set. Serve hot.

17. Chia Seed Breakfast Pudding:

- *Ingredients:*

- 1/4 cup chia seeds

- 1 cup almond milk

- 1 tablespoon maple syrup

- 1/2 teaspoon vanilla extract

- Sliced strawberries for topping

- ### *Instructions:*

1.   In a bowl or jar, mix chia seeds, almond milk, maple syrup, and vanilla extract. Stir well, cover, and refrigerate for at least 2 hours or overnight, until thickened.

2.   Serve topped with sliced strawberries before serving.

18. *Egg and Avocado Toast:*

- ### *Ingredients:*

  - 1 slice whole grain bread, toasted

  - 1/2 avocado, mashed

  - 1 hard-boiled egg, sliced

  - Pinch of red pepper flakes

  - Drizzle of olive oil

- ### *Instructions:*

1.   Spread mashed avocado on the toasted whole grain bread.

2.   Top with sliced hard-boiled egg, red pepper flakes, and a drizzle of olive oil before serving.

19. *Raspberry Coconut Smoothie:*

- Ingredients:

  - 1/2 cup raspberries

- 1/4 cup coconut milk

- 1/2 banana

- 1/2 cup Greek yogurt

- 1 tablespoon honey or maple syrup

- *Instructions:*

1. Blend raspberries, coconut milk, banana, Greek yogurt, and honey or maple syrup until smooth.

2. Serve immediately.

20. Tomato and Basil Breakfast Frittata:

- *Ingredients:*

  - 4 eggs

  - 1/4 cup cherry tomatoes, halved

  - 1 tablespoon chopped fresh basil

  - 1 tablespoon grated Parmesan cheese

  - Salt and pepper to taste

- *Instructions:*

1. Preheat oven to 350°F (175°C). In a bowl, beat the eggs and season with salt and pepper.

2. Pour the beaten eggs into a greased oven-safe skillet.

3. Sprinkle cherry tomatoes, chopped basil, and grated Parmesan cheese evenly over the eggs.

4. Bake for 12-15 minutes, or until the eggs are set. Slice into wedges and serve hot.

21. Chocolate Peanut Butter Smoothie:

- *Ingredients:*

- 1 cup unsweetened almond milk

- 1 banana

- 2 tablespoons unsweetened cocoa powder

- 2 tablespoons natural peanut butter

- 1 tablespoon honey or maple syrup

- *Instructions:*

1. Blend almond milk, banana, cocoa powder, peanut butter, and honey or maple syrup until smooth.

2. Serve chilled.

22. Blueberry Almond Butter Overnight Oats:

- *Ingredients:*

  - 1/2 cup rolled oats

  - 1/2 cup almond milk

  - 1/4 cup blueberries

  - 2 tablespoons almond butter

  - 1 tablespoon honey or maple syrup

- *Instructions:*

1. In a jar or container, combine rolled oats, almond milk, blueberries, almond butter, and honey or maple syrup. Stir well, cover, and refrigerate overnight. Enjoy cold in the morning.

23. Egg White Veggie Scramble:

- *Ingredients:*

- 4 egg whites

- 1/4 cup diced bell peppers

- 1/4 cup diced zucchini

- 1/4 cup diced tomatoes

- 1 tablespoon chopped parsley

- Salt and pepper to taste

- *Instructions:*

1. In a skillet, sauté diced bell peppers, zucchini, and tomatoes until tender.

2. Add egg whites to the skillet and cook, stirring occasionally, until scrambled.

3. Season with salt, pepper, and chopped parsley before serving.

24. Coconut Mango Chia Pudding:

- *Ingredients:*

  - 1/4 cup chia seeds

  - 1 cup coconut milk

  - 1/2 cup diced mango

  - 1 tablespoon honey or maple syrup

  - Shredded coconut for garnish

- *Instructions:*

1. In a bowl or jar, mix chia seeds, coconut milk, diced mango, and honey or maple syrup. Stir well, cover, and refrigerate for at least 2 hours or overnight, until thickened. Serve chilled, topped with shredded coconut.

25. Spinach and Mushroom Breakfast Quesadilla:

- *Ingredients:*

  - 1 whole grain tortilla

  - 1/2 cup baby spinach

  - 1/4 cup sliced mushrooms

  - 1/4 cup shredded mozzarella cheese

  - 1 tablespoon salsa

- *Instructions:*

1. Heat a skillet over medium heat and place the tortilla in the skillet.

2. Layer one half of the tortilla with baby spinach, sliced mushrooms, and shredded mozzarella cheese. Fold the other half over the toppings to form a quesadilla.

3. Cook for 2-3 minutes on each side, or until the tortilla is golden brown and the cheese is melted. Serve hot with salsa.

26. Peaches and Cream Overnight Oats:

- *Ingredients:*

  - 1/2 cup rolled oats

  - 1/2 cup almond milk

  - 1/2 ripe peach, diced

  - 2 tablespoons Greek yogurt

  - 1 tablespoon honey or maple syrup

- *Instructions:*

1. In a jar or container, combine rolled oats, almond milk, diced peach, Greek yogurt, and honey or maple syrup. Stir well, cover, and refrigerate overnight. Enjoy cold in the morning.

27. Broccoli and Cheddar Egg Muffins:

- *Ingredients:*

  - 4 large eggs

  - 1/2 cup chopped broccoli florets

  - 1/4 cup shredded cheddar cheese

  - 1 tablespoon chopped chives

  - Salt and pepper to taste

- *Instructions:*

1. Preheat oven to 350°F (175°C). In a bowl, whisk together eggs, chopped broccoli florets, shredded cheddar cheese, chopped chives, salt, and pepper.

2. Pour mixture into greased muffin tins, filling each cup 3/4 full. Bake for 20-25 minutes, or until eggs are set. Allow to cool slightly before serving.

28. Peanut Butter Banana Breakfast Wrap:

- *Ingredients:*

  - 1 whole grain wrap or tortilla

  - 2 tablespoons peanut butter

  - 1 banana, sliced

  - Drizzle of honey

- *Instructions:*

1. Spread peanut butter on the whole grain wrap.

2. Arrange banana slices on top of the peanut butter and drizzle with honey. Roll up tightly before serving.

29. Cherry Almond Smoothie:

- **Ingredients:**

    - 1/2 cup frozen cherries

    - 1/2 banana

    - 1/4 cup almond milk

    - 1/4 cup Greek yogurt

    - 1 tablespoon almond butter

    - 1 teaspoon honey or maple syrup

- **Instructions:**

1.   Blend frozen cherries, banana, almond milk, Greek yogurt, almond butter, and honey or maple syrup until smooth. Serve immediately.

30. Tomato Basil Avocado Toast:

- **Ingredients:**

    - 1 slice whole grain bread, toasted

    - 1/4 ripe avocado, mashed

    - 2 slices tomato

    - 2 fresh basil leaves

    - Drizzle of balsamic glaze

- **Instructions:**

1.   Spread mashed avocado on the toasted whole grain bread.

2.   Top with tomato slices, fresh basil leaves, and a drizzle of balsamic glaze before serving.

31. Pumpkin Spice Smoothie:

- Ingredients:

    - 1/2 cup pumpkin puree

    - 1/2 banana

    - 1/2 cup almond milk

    - 1/4 teaspoon pumpkin pie spice

    - 1 tablespoon honey or maple syrup

    - Ice cubes (optional)

- Instructions:

1. Blend pumpkin puree, banana, almond milk, pumpkin pie spice, honey or maple syrup, and ice cubes until smooth. Serve chilled.

These recipes offer a variety of flavors and nutrients to help you kick-start your day on a healthy note. Enjoy experimenting with different ingredients and combinations!

CHAPTER 3: LUNCH

1. Grilled Chicken Salad:

- ### Ingredients:

    - 4 oz grilled chicken breast, sliced

    - 2 cups mixed salad greens

    - 1/4 cup cherry tomatoes, halved

    - 1/4 cucumber, sliced

    - 1/4 avocado, diced

    - 1 tablespoon balsamic vinaigrette

- ### Instructions:

1. Arrange salad greens on a plate.

2. Top with grilled chicken slices, cherry tomatoes, cucumber, and avocado.

3. Drizzle with balsamic vinaigrette before serving.

2. Quinoa Stuffed Bell Peppers:

- ### Ingredients:

    - 2 bell peppers, halved and seeded

    - 1/2 cup cooked quinoa

    - 1/4 cup black beans, drained and rinsed

    - 1/4 cup corn kernels

    - 1/4 cup diced tomatoes

    - 1/4 cup shredded cheddar cheese

- 1 teaspoon taco seasoning

- *Instructions:*

  1. Preheat oven to 375°F (190°C).

  2. In a bowl, mix cooked quinoa, black beans, corn, diced tomatoes, shredded cheddar cheese, and taco seasoning.

  3. Stuff each bell pepper half with the quinoa mixture.

  4. Place stuffed bell peppers on a baking sheet and bake for 20-25 minutes, or until peppers are tender.

3. Salmon and Asparagus Foil Packets:

- *Ingredients*:

  - 4 oz salmon fillet

  - 6 spears asparagus

  - 1/4 lemon, sliced

  - 1 tablespoon olive oil

  - Salt and pepper to taste

- *Instructions:*

  1. Preheat oven to 400°F (200°C).

  2. Place each salmon fillet on a piece of aluminum foil.

  3. Arrange asparagus spears around the salmon.

  4. Drizzle salmon and asparagus with olive oil and season with salt and pepper.

  5. Place lemon slices on top of the salmon.

  6. Fold the foil over the salmon and seal tightly.

7. Bake for 15-20 minutes, or until salmon is cooked through and asparagus is tender. And serve.

4. Mediterranean Chickpea Salad:

- **Ingredients:**

  - 1 can (15 oz) chickpeas, drained and rinsed

  - 1/2 cucumber, diced

  - 1/2 cup cherry tomatoes, halved

  - 1/4 cup diced red onion

  - 2 tablespoons chopped fresh parsley

  - 2 tablespoons crumbled feta cheese

  - 1 tablespoon olive oil

  - 1 tablespoon lemon juice

  - Salt and pepper to taste

- **Instructions:**

  1. In a large bowl, combine chickpeas, cucumber, cherry tomatoes, red onion, parsley, and feta cheese.

  2. Drizzle olive oil and lemon juice over the salad.

  3. Season with salt and pepper, toss to combine, and serve chilled.

5. Turkey and Hummus Wrap:

- **Ingredients:**

  - 4 oz sliced turkey breast

  - 1 whole grain wrap or tortilla

- 2 tablespoons hummus

- 1/4 cup baby spinach leaves

- 1/4 cup shredded carrots

- 1/4 avocado, sliced

- *Instructions:*

    1. Spread hummus evenly over the whole grain wrap.

    2. Layer sliced turkey breast, baby spinach leaves, shredded carrots, and avocado slices on the wrap.

    3. Roll up tightly and slice in half before serving.

6. Veggie Stir-Fry with Tofu:

- *Ingredients:*

    - 1/2 block (7 oz) firm tofu, cubed

    - 1 cup mixed stir-fry vegetables (bell peppers, broccoli, snap peas)

    - 1 tablespoon soy sauce

    - 1 tablespoon hoisin sauce

    - 1 teaspoon sesame oil

    - 1/2 teaspoon minced garlic

    - Cooked brown rice for serving

- *Instructions:*

    1. Heat sesame oil in a skillet over medium heat.

    2. Add cubed tofu and stir-fry until lightly browned.

3. Add mixed vegetables and minced garlic to the skillet. Cook until vegetables are tender-crisp.

4. Stir in soy sauce and hoisin sauce, and cook for an additional minute.

5. Serve stir-fry over cooked brown rice.

7. Caprese Pasta Salad:

- ### *Ingredients:*

  - 1 cup cooked whole wheat pasta

  - 1/2 cup cherry tomatoes, halved

  - 1/2 cup fresh mozzarella balls

  - 2 tablespoons chopped fresh basil

  - 1 tablespoon balsamic glaze

  - Salt and pepper to taste

- ### *Instructions:*

  1. In a bowl, combine cooked pasta, cherry tomatoes, fresh mozzarella balls, and chopped fresh basil.

  2. Drizzle with balsamic glaze and season with salt and pepper.

  3. Toss to combine and serve chilled.

8. Lentil and Vegetable Soup:

- ### *Ingredients:*

  - 1/2 cup dried lentils, rinsed

  - 1 carrot, diced

  - 1 celery stalk, diced

- 1/4 onion, diced

- 2 cups vegetable broth

- 1/2 teaspoon dried thyme

- Salt and pepper to taste

- *Instructions:*

  1. In a pot, combine dried lentils, diced carrot, celery, onion, vegetable broth, and dried thyme.

  2. Bring to a boil, then reduce heat and simmer for 20-25 minutes, or until lentils are tender.

  3. Season with salt and pepper before serving.

9. Tuna Salad Stuffed Avocado:

- *Ingredients:*

  - 1 ripe avocado, halved and pitted

  - 1 can (5 oz) tuna, drained

  - 1 tablespoon Greek yogurt

  - 1 tablespoon diced red onion

  - 1 tablespoon chopped fresh parsley

  - 1 teaspoon Dijon mustard

  - Salt and pepper to taste

- *Instructions:*

  1. In a bowl, mix tuna, Greek yogurt, diced red onion, chopped parsley, Dijon mustard, salt, and pepper.

  2. Spoon tuna salad into the halved avocado.

3. Serve immediately.

10. Mango Chicken Lettuce Wraps:

- ### Ingredients:

  - 4 oz cooked chicken breast, shredded

  - 1/2 mango, diced

  - 1/4 red bell pepper, diced

  - 2 tablespoons chopped cilantro

  - 1 tablespoon lime juice

  - 1 teaspoon honey

  - Butter lettuce leaves for wrapping

- ### Instructions:

  1. In a bowl, combine shredded chicken, diced mango, diced red bell pepper, chopped cilantro, lime juice, and honey.

  2. Spoon the chicken mixture onto butter lettuce leaves.

  3. Roll up the leaves and secure with toothpicks before serving.

11. Cucumber and Hummus Sandwich:

- ### Ingredients:

  - 2 slices whole grain bread

  - 2 tablespoons hummus

  - 4 cucumber slices

  - 2 slices tomato

  - 1/4 avocado, mashed

- Salt and pepper to taste

- *Instructions:*

  1. Spread hummus on one slice of whole grain bread.

  2. Layer cucumber slices and tomato slices on top.

  3. Spread mashed avocado on the other slice of bread and place it on top of the sandwich.

  4. Season with salt and pepper, then slice in half before serving.

12. Miso Glazed Salmon Salad:

- *Ingredients:*

  - 4 oz salmon fillet

  - 2 cups mixed salad greens

  - 1/4 cup shredded carrots

  - 1/4 cup sliced cucumber

  - 1 tablespoon miso paste

  - 1 tablespoon soy sauce

  - 1 tablespoon honey

  - 1 teaspoon sesame oil

- *Instructions:*

  1. Preheat oven to 400°F (200°C).

  2. In a small bowl, mix miso paste, soy sauce, honey, and sesame oil.

  3. Place salmon fillet on a baking sheet and brush with the miso glaze.

  4. Bake for 12-15 minutes, or until salmon is cooked through.

5. Arrange salad greens, shredded carrots, and sliced cucumber on a plate.

6. Top with cooked miso glazed salmon before serving.

13. Pesto Chicken Pasta Salad:

- **Ingredients:**

  - 1 cup cooked whole wheat pasta

  - 4 oz cooked chicken breast, diced

  - 2 tablespoons pesto sauce

  - 1/4 cup cherry tomatoes, halved

  - 1/4 cup diced cucumber

  - 1/4 cup sliced black olives

- **Instructions:**

  1. In a bowl, combine cooked pasta, diced chicken breast, pesto sauce, cherry tomatoes, diced cucumber, and sliced black olives.

  2. Toss to combine and serve chilled.

14. Eggplant and Tomato Stack:

- **Ingredients:**

  - 1 small eggplant, sliced into rounds

  - 1 large tomato, sliced

  - 2 tablespoons olive oil

  - 1 teaspoon Italian seasoning

  - Salt and pepper to taste

  - 2 tablespoons balsamic glaze

- Fresh basil leaves for garnish

- *Instructions:*

  1. Preheat oven to 400°F (200°C).

  2. Arrange eggplant slices on a baking sheet and brush with olive oil.

  3. Season with Italian seasoning, salt, and pepper.

  4. Roast in the oven for 15-20 minutes, or until eggplant is tender.

  5. Remove from the oven and let cool slightly.

  6. To assemble, layer eggplant slices with tomato slices.

  7. Drizzle with balsamic glaze and garnish with fresh basil leaves before serving.

15. Turkey and Vegetable Lettuce Wraps:

- *Ingredients:*

  - 4 large lettuce leaves (such as romaine or butter lettuce)

  - 4 oz sliced turkey breast

  - 1/4 cup shredded carrots

  - 1/4 cup sliced bell peppers

  - 1/4 cup sliced cucumber

  - 2 tablespoons hummus

- *Instructions:*

  1. Lay lettuce leaves flat on a plate.

  2. Top each lettuce leaf with sliced turkey breast, shredded carrots, sliced bell peppers, and sliced cucumber.

  3. Spread hummus over the toppings.

4. Roll up the lettuce leaves and secure with toothpicks before serving.

16. Black Bean and Corn Salad:

- *Ingredients:*

  - 1 can (15 oz) black beans, drained and rinsed
  - 1 cup corn kernels (fresh, frozen, or canned)
  - 1/4 cup diced red onion
  - 1/4 cup chopped fresh cilantro
  - 1 tablespoon olive oil
  - 1 tablespoon lime juice
  - Salt and pepper to taste

- *Instructions:*

  1. In a bowl, combine black beans, corn kernels, diced red onion, and chopped fresh cilantro.
  2. Drizzle with olive oil and lime juice.
  3. Season with salt and pepper, toss to combine, and serve chilled.

17. Shrimp and Vegetable Stir-Fry:

- *Ingredients:*

  - 4 oz shrimp, peeled and deveined
  - 1 cup mixed stir-fry vegetables (bell peppers, broccoli, snap peas)
  - 1 tablespoon soy sauce
  - 1 tablespoon oyster sauce
  - 1 teaspoon sesame oil

- 1/2 teaspoon minced garlic

- Cooked brown rice for serving

- *Instructions:*

    1. Heat sesame oil in a skillet over medium heat.

    2. Add shrimp and minced garlic to the skillet. Cook until shrimp turns pink.

    3. Add mixed vegetables to the skillet and stir-fry until tender-crisp.

    4. Stir in soy sauce and oyster sauce, and cook for an additional minute.

    5. Serve stir-fry over cooked brown rice.

18. Cauliflower Rice Sushi Rolls:

- *Ingredients:*

    - 2 nori seaweed sheets

    - 1 cup cauliflower rice

    - 4 oz cooked crab meat or imitation crab sticks

    - 1/4 avocado, sliced

    - 1/4 cucumber, julienned

    - 1 tablespoon rice vinegar

    - Soy sauce and wasabi for dipping

- *Instructions:*

    1. Place nori seaweed sheets on a clean surface.

    2. Spread cauliflower rice evenly over each sheet, leaving a small border along the edges.

    3. Top with cooked crab meat, avocado slices, and julienned cucumber.

4. Sprinkle rice vinegar over the toppings.

5. Roll up the nori sheets tightly, then slice into bite-sized pieces.

6. Serve with soy sauce and wasabi for dipping.

19. Mushroom and Spinach Quesadillas:

- ### Ingredients:

  - 2 whole grain tortillas

  - 1 cup sliced mushrooms

  - 1 cup baby spinach leaves

  - 1/2 cup shredded mozzarella cheese

  - 2 tablespoons salsa

  - Cooking spray

- ### Instructions:

  1. Heat a skillet over medium heat and coat with cooking spray.

  2. Place one tortilla in the skillet and sprinkle half of the shredded mozzarella cheese over it.

  3. Top with sliced mushrooms, baby spinach leaves, and salsa.

  4. Sprinkle the remaining shredded mozzarella cheese over the toppings.

  5. Place the second tortilla on top and press down gently.

  6. Cook for 2-3 minutes on each side, or until the tortillas are golden brown and the cheese is melted.

  7. Slice into wedges and serve warm.

20. Greek Chickpea Salad:

- *Ingredients:*

    - 1 can (15 oz) chickpeas, drained and rinsed

    - 1/2 cucumber, diced

    - 1/2 cup cherry tomatoes, halved

    - 1/4 cup diced red onion

    - 1/4 cup crumbled feta cheese

    - 2 tablespoons chopped fresh parsley

    - 1 tablespoon olive oil

    - 1 tablespoon lemon juice

    - Salt and pepper to taste

- *Instructions:*

    1. In a large bowl, combine chickpeas, cucumber, cherry tomatoes, red onion, feta cheese, and chopped fresh parsley.

    2. Drizzle olive oil and lemon juice over the salad.

    3. Season with salt and pepper, toss to combine, and serve chilled.

21. Turkey and Veggie Lettuce Wraps:

- *Ingredients:*

    - 4 large lettuce leaves (such as romaine or butter lettuce)

    - 4 oz sliced turkey breast

    - 1/4 cup shredded carrots

    - 1/4 cup sliced bell peppers

    - 1/4 cup sliced cucumber

- 2 tablespoons hummus

- *Instructions:*

  1. Lay lettuce leaves flat on a plate.

  2. Top each lettuce leaf with sliced turkey breast, shredded carrots, sliced bell peppers, and sliced cucumber.

  3. Spread hummus over the toppings.

  4. Roll up the lettuce leaves and secure with toothpicks before serving.

22. Quinoa Salad with Roasted Vegetables:

- *Ingredients:*

  - 1/2 cup cooked quinoa

  - 1/2 cup roasted vegetables (such as bell peppers, zucchini, and eggplant)

  - 1/4 cup cherry tomatoes, halved

  - 2 tablespoons crumbled feta cheese

  - 1 tablespoon chopped fresh parsley

  - 1 tablespoon balsamic vinaigrette

- *Instructions:*

  1. In a bowl, combine cooked quinoa, roasted vegetables, cherry tomatoes, crumbled feta cheese, and chopped fresh parsley.

  2. Drizzle with balsamic vinaigrette and toss to combine.

  3. Serve chilled or at room temperature.

23. Miso Glazed Tofu Stir-Fry:

- *Ingredients:*

- 1/2 block (7 oz) firm tofu, cubed

- 1 cup mixed stir-fry vegetables (bell peppers, broccoli, snap peas)

- 1 tablespoon soy sauce

- 1 tablespoon miso paste

- 1 teaspoon sesame oil

- 1/2 teaspoon minced garlic

- Cooked brown rice for serving

- *Instructions:*

1. Heat sesame oil in a skillet over medium heat.

2. Add cubed tofu and minced garlic to the skillet. Cook until tofu is lightly browned.

3. Add mixed vegetables to the skillet and stir-fry until tender-crisp.

4. In a small bowl, mix soy sauce and miso paste. Pour over the tofu and vegetables, and stir to combine.

5. Cook for an additional minute, then serve stir-fry over cooked brown rice.

24. Tomato Basil Mozzarella Panini:

- *Ingredients:*

    - 2 slices whole grain bread

    - 2 slices fresh mozzarella cheese

    - 2 slices tomato

    - 2 fresh basil leaves

    - 1 teaspoon balsamic glaze

    - Cooking spray

- *Instructions:*

    1. Heat a panini press or skillet over medium heat and coat with cooking spray.

    2. Place one slice of whole grain bread on the panini press or skillet.

    3. Layer fresh mozzarella cheese slices, tomato slices, and fresh basil leaves on top.

    4. Drizzle with balsamic glaze, then top with the second slice of whole grain bread.

    5. Cook in the panini press or skillet until the bread is toasted and the cheese is melted.

    6. Slice in half and serve warm.

25. Tofu and Vegetable Curry:

- *Ingredients:*

    - 1/2 block (7 oz) firm tofu, cubed

    - 1 cup mixed vegetables (such as bell peppers, carrots, and broccoli)

    - 1/2 cup coconut milk

    - 2 tablespoons red curry paste

    - 1 tablespoon soy sauce

    - 1 tablespoon maple syrup

    - Cooked brown rice for serving

- Instructions:

    1. In a saucepan, combine coconut milk, red curry paste, soy sauce, and maple syrup.

    2. Bring to a simmer over medium heat.

    3. Add cubed tofu and mixed vegetables to the saucepan.

4. Simmer for 10-12 minutes, or until vegetables are tender and tofu is heated through.

5. Serve curry over cooked brown rice.

26. Mediterranean Tuna Salad:

- *Ingredients:*

  - 1 can (5 oz) tuna, drained

  - 1/4 cup diced cucumber

  - 1/4 cup cherry tomatoes, halved

  - 2 tablespoons diced red onion

  - 2 tablespoons chopped Kalamata olives

  - 1 tablespoon chopped fresh parsley

  - 1 tablespoon olive oil

  - 1 tablespoon lemon juice

  - Salt and pepper to taste

- *Instructions:*

  1. In a bowl, combine drained tuna, diced cucumber, cherry tomatoes, diced red onion, Kalamata olives, and chopped fresh parsley.

  2. Drizzle with olive oil and lemon juice.

  3. Season with salt and pepper, toss to combine, and serve chilled.

27. Sesame Ginger Tofu Salad:

- *Ingredients:*

  - 1/2 block (7 oz) firm tofu, cubed

- 2 cups mixed salad greens

- 1/4 cup shredded carrots

- 1/4 cup sliced cucumber

- 1/4 cup sliced red bell pepper

- 2 tablespoons sliced almonds

- 1 tablespoon sesame seeds

- 2 tablespoons sesame ginger dressing

- *Instructions:*

  1. Heat a skillet over medium heat and add cubed tofu.

  2. Cook until tofu is lightly browned and heated through.

  3. In a large bowl, combine mixed salad greens, shredded carrots, sliced cucumber, sliced red bell pepper, sliced almonds, and sesame seeds.

  4. Add cooked tofu to the salad, drizzle with sesame ginger dressing, and toss to combine.

  5. Serve immediately.

28. Mushroom and Spinach Flatbread Pizza:

- *Ingredients:*

  - 1 whole grain flatbread

  - 1/2 cup sliced mushrooms

  - 1 cup baby spinach leaves

  - 1/4 cup shredded mozzarella cheese

  - 1 tablespoon tomato sauce

  - 1/2 teaspoon dried oregano

- 1/2 teaspoon crushed red pepper flakes

- *Instructions:*

   1. Preheat oven to 400°F (200°C).

   2. Spread tomato sauce evenly over the whole grain flatbread.

   3. Top with sliced mushrooms, baby spinach leaves, and shredded mozzarella cheese.

   4. Sprinkle dried oregano and crushed red pepper flakes over the toppings.

   5. Place the flatbread on a baking sheet and bake for 10-12 minutes, or until cheese is melted and bubbly.

   6. Slice into wedges and serve hot.

29. Chicken Caesar Salad Wrap:

- *Ingredients:*

   - 4 oz grilled chicken breast, sliced

   - 1 whole grain wrap or tortilla

   - 1/4 cup chopped romaine lettuce

   - 2 tablespoons Caesar dressing

   - 1 tablespoon grated Parmesan cheese

   - Salt and pepper to taste

- *Instructions:*

   1. Spread Caesar dressing evenly over the whole grain wrap.

   2. Layer sliced grilled chicken breast and chopped romaine lettuce on the wrap.

   3. Sprinkle grated Parmesan cheese over the toppings.

4. Season with salt and pepper, then roll up tightly and slice in half before serving.

30. Asian Noodle Salad:

- *Ingredients:*

    - 1 cup cooked soba noodles

    - 1/2 cup shredded cabbage

    - 1/4 cup shredded carrots

    - 1/4 cup edamame

    - 2 tablespoons sliced green onions

    - 1 tablespoon sesame oil

    - 1 tablespoon soy sauce

    - 1 tablespoon rice vinegar

    - 1/2 teaspoon grated ginger

    - Sesame seeds for garnish

- *Instructions:*

    1. In a bowl, combine cooked soba noodles, shredded cabbage, shredded carrots, edamame, and sliced green onions.

    2. In a small bowl, whisk together sesame oil, soy sauce, rice vinegar, and grated ginger.

    3. Pour the dressing over the noodle mixture and toss to combine.

    4. Garnish with sesame seeds before serving.

31. Turkey and White Bean Chili:

- *Ingredients:*

- 1 lb ground turkey

- 1 can (15 oz) white beans, drained and rinsed

- 1 can (14.5 oz) diced tomatoes

- 1 cup low-sodium chicken broth

- 1/2 onion, diced

- 2 cloves garlic, minced

- 1 teaspoon chili powder

- 1/2 teaspoon ground cumin

- Salt and pepper to taste

- Chopped fresh cilantro for garnish

- ***Instructions:***

   1. In a large pot, cook ground turkey over medium heat until browned.

   2. Add diced onion and minced garlic to the pot. Cook until onion is translucent.

   3. Stir in white beans, diced tomatoes, chicken broth, chili powder, and ground cumin.

   4. Bring to a simmer and cook for 15-20 minutes, stirring occasionally.

   5. Season with salt and pepper to taste.

   6. Serve hot, garnished with chopped fresh cilantro.

These recipes provide a variety of flavorful and nutritious options for cancer-friendly lunches. Enjoy experimenting with different ingredients and flavors!

CHAPTER 4: DINNER

1. Grilled Lemon Herb Chicken:

- ### Ingredients:

    - 4 boneless, skinless chicken breasts
    - 2 tablespoons olive oil
    - 2 cloves garlic, minced
    - Zest and juice of 1 lemon
    - 1 teaspoon dried thyme
    - 1 teaspoon dried rosemary
    - Salt and pepper to taste

- ### Instructions:

1. In a bowl, mix olive oil, minced garlic, lemon zest, lemon juice, dried thyme, dried rosemary, salt, and pepper.

2. Add chicken breasts to the bowl and coat them with the marinade. Let marinate in the refrigerator for at least 30 minutes.

3. Preheat grill to medium-high heat. Grill chicken breasts for 6-8 minutes per side, or until cooked through.

4. Serve hot with your choice of sides.

2. Baked Lemon Garlic Salmon:

- ### Ingredients:

    - 4 salmon fillets (4-6 oz each)
    - 2 tablespoons olive oil

- 2 cloves garlic, minced

- Zest and juice of 1 lemon

- 1 teaspoon dried oregano

- Salt and pepper to taste

- *Instructions:*

1. Preheat oven to 375°F (190°C). Line a baking sheet with parchment paper.

2. Place salmon fillets on the prepared baking sheet.

3. In a small bowl, mix olive oil, minced garlic, lemon zest, lemon juice, dried oregano, salt, and pepper.

4. Drizzle the olive oil mixture over the salmon fillets.

5. Bake for 12-15 minutes, or until salmon is cooked through and flakes easily with a fork.

6. Serve hot with your favorite vegetables or salad.

3. Quinoa and Black Bean Stuffed Peppers:

- *Ingredients:*

- 4 bell peppers, halved and seeds removed

- 1 cup cooked quinoa

- 1 cup black beans, drained and rinsed

- 1 cup corn kernels

- 1 cup diced tomatoes

- 1 teaspoon chili powder

- 1/2 teaspoon cumin

- Salt and pepper to taste

- Grated cheese for topping (optional)

- ***Instructions:***

  1. Preheat oven to 375°F (190°C). Place halved bell peppers in a baking dish.

  2. In a large bowl, combine cooked quinoa, black beans, corn kernels, diced tomatoes, chili powder, cumin, salt, and pepper.

  3. Spoon the quinoa and black bean mixture into each bell pepper half.

  4. Top each stuffed pepper with grated cheese if desired.

  5. Cover the baking dish with foil and bake for 25-30 minutes, or until peppers are tender.

  6. Serve hot with a side of avocado or salsa.

4. Mediterranean Chickpea Salad:

- ***Ingredients:***

  - 2 cups cooked chickpeas (or 1 can, drained and rinsed)

  - 1 cucumber, diced

  - 1 cup cherry tomatoes, halved

  - 1/2 red onion, thinly sliced

  - 1/4 cup Kalamata olives, pitted and halved

  - 1/4 cup crumbled feta cheese

  - 2 tablespoons chopped fresh parsley

  - 2 tablespoons olive oil

  - 1 tablespoon lemon juice

  - 1 teaspoon dried oregano

  - Salt and pepper to taste

- *Instructions:*

    1. In a large bowl, combine cooked chickpeas, diced cucumber, halved cherry tomatoes, thinly sliced red onion, halved Kalamata olives, crumbled feta cheese, and chopped fresh parsley.

    2. In a small bowl, whisk together olive oil, lemon juice, dried oregano, salt, and pepper.

    3. Drizzle the dressing over the chickpea salad and toss to combine.

    4. Serve chilled or at room temperature as a main dish or side salad.

5. Grilled Vegetable Quinoa Bowl:

- *Ingredients:*

    - 1 cup cooked quinoa

    - 2 cups mixed grilled vegetables (such as zucchini, bell peppers, eggplant, and mushrooms), chopped

    - 1/4 cup crumbled feta cheese

    - 2 tablespoons chopped fresh basil

    - 2 tablespoons balsamic glaze

    - Salt and pepper to taste

- *Instructions:*

    1. In a bowl, combine cooked quinoa and mixed grilled vegetables.

    2. Sprinkle crumbled feta cheese and chopped fresh basil over the quinoa and vegetable mixture.

    3. Drizzle balsamic glaze over the bowl and season with salt and pepper to taste.

    4. Serve warm or at room temperature as a nutritious and filling dinner option.

6. Turkey and Vegetable Stir-Fry:

- ### Ingredients:

  - 1 lb turkey breast, thinly sliced

  - 2 tablespoons soy sauce

  - 1 tablespoon hoisin sauce

  - 1 tablespoon sesame oil

  - 2 cloves garlic, minced

  - 1 teaspoon grated ginger

  - 2 cups mixed vegetables (such as broccoli, carrots, bell peppers, and snap peas), sliced

  - Cooked brown rice for serving

  - Chopped green onions for garnish

- ### Instructions:

  1. In a bowl, toss thinly sliced turkey breast with soy sauce and hoisin sauce.

  2. Heat sesame oil in a large skillet or wok over medium-high heat. Add minced garlic and grated ginger, and cook for 1 minute.

  3. Add turkey slices to the skillet and stir-fry until cooked through.

  4. Add mixed vegetables to the skillet and stir-fry until tender-crisp.

  5. Serve turkey and vegetable stir-fry over cooked brown rice.

  6. Garnish with chopped green onions before serving.

7. Lentil and Vegetable Curry:

- ### Ingredients:

- 1 cup dried green lentils, rinsed

- 2 cups vegetable broth

- 1 tablespoon olive oil

- 1 onion, diced

- 2 cloves garlic, minced

- 1 tablespoon grated ginger

- 2 tablespoons curry powder

- 1 teaspoon ground cumin

- 1 teaspoon ground turmeric

- 1 can (14 oz) diced tomatoes

- 2 cups mixed vegetables (such as cauliflower, carrots, and peas)

- 1 can (14 oz) coconut milk

- Salt and pepper to taste

- Chopped fresh cilantro for garnish

- ***Instructions:***

1. In a saucepan, combine rinsed green lentils and vegetable broth. Bring to a boil, then reduce heat and simmer for 20-25 minutes, or until lentils are tender.

2. In a large skillet, heat olive oil over medium heat. Add diced onion and cook until softened.

3. Add minced garlic, grated ginger, curry powder, ground cumin, and ground turmeric to the skillet. Cook for 1-2 minutes, until fragrant.

4. Stir in diced tomatoes (with their juices) and mixed vegetables. Cook for 5-7 minutes, until vegetables are tender.

5. Add cooked lentils and coconut milk to the skillet. Stir well to combine.

6. Simmer curry for an additional 5-10 minutes to allow flavors to meld. Season with salt and pepper to taste.

7. Serve hot over cooked rice or quinoa, garnished with chopped fresh cilantro.

8. *Honey Garlic Shrimp Stir-Fry:*

- ## *Ingredients:*

  - 1 lb shrimp, peeled and deveined

  - 2 tablespoons olive oil

  - 4 cloves garlic, minced

  - 1 tablespoon grated ginger

  - 2 tablespoons honey

  - 3 tablespoons soy sauce

  - 2 cups mixed vegetables (such as bell peppers, snap peas, and broccoli), sliced

  - Cooked brown rice or noodles for serving

  - Sesame seeds for garnish

- ## *Instructions:*

  1. In a bowl, toss peeled and deveined shrimp with minced garlic, grated ginger, honey, and soy sauce. Let marinate for 15-20 minutes.

  2. Heat olive oil in a large skillet or wok over medium-high heat. Add marinated shrimp to the skillet and cook for 2-3 minutes on each side, until pink and cooked through. Remove shrimp from the skillet and set aside.

  3. In the same skillet, add sliced mixed vegetables and stir-fry until tender-crisp.

  4. Return cooked shrimp to the skillet and toss with the vegetables.

  5. Serve honey garlic shrimp stir-fry over cooked brown rice or noodles.

6. Garnish with sesame seeds before serving.

9. Caprese Stuffed Chicken Breast:

- *Ingredients:*

  - 4 boneless, skinless chicken breasts

  - 1 cup cherry tomatoes, halved

  - 4 slices mozzarella cheese

  - 1/4 cup fresh basil leaves

  - 2 tablespoons balsamic glaze

  - Salt and pepper to taste

- *Instructions:*

  1. Preheat oven to 400°F (200°C). Line a baking sheet with parchment paper.

  2. Place chicken breasts on the prepared baking sheet. Using a sharp knife, cut a slit in the side of each chicken breast to create a pocket.

  3. Stuff each chicken breast with halved cherry tomatoes, a slice of mozzarella cheese, and fresh basil leaves.

  4. Season stuffed chicken breasts with salt and pepper.

  5. Bake for 25-30 minutes, or until chicken is cooked through and no longer pink in the center.

  6. Drizzle balsamic glaze over the stuffed chicken breasts before serving.

10. Tofu and Vegetable Stir-Fry:

- *Ingredients:*

  - 1 block (14 oz) firm tofu, drained and cubed

- 2 tablespoons soy sauce

- 1 tablespoon sesame oil

- 2 cloves garlic, minced

- 1 teaspoon grated ginger

- 2 cups mixed vegetables (such as bell peppers, broccoli, and carrots), sliced

- Cooked brown rice for serving

- Chopped green onions for garnish

- ### *Instructions:*

  1. In a bowl, toss cubed tofu with soy sauce and sesame oil.

  2. Heat a large skillet or wok over medium-high heat. Add tofu cubes and cook until golden brown on all sides. Remove tofu from the skillet and set aside.

  3. In the same skillet, add minced garlic and grated ginger. Cook for 1 minute.

  4. Add mixed vegetables to the skillet and stir-fry until tender-crisp.

  5. Return cooked tofu to the skillet and toss with the vegetables.

  6. Serve tofu and vegetable stir-fry over cooked brown rice.

  7. Garnish with chopped green onions before serving.

11. Lemon Garlic Shrimp Pasta:

- ### *Ingredients:*

  - 8 oz whole wheat spaghetti

  - 1 lb shrimp, peeled and deveined

  - 2 tablespoons olive oil

  - 4 cloves garlic, minced

- Zest and juice of 1 lemon

- 1/4 teaspoon red pepper flakes

- Salt and pepper to taste

- Chopped fresh parsley for garnish

- *Instructions:*

1. Cook whole wheat spaghetti according to package instructions until al dente. Drain and set aside.

2. In a large skillet, heat olive oil over medium heat. Add minced garlic and cook until fragrant.

3. Add shrimp to the skillet and cook for 2-3 minutes on each side, until pink and cooked through.

4. Stir in lemon zest, lemon juice, red pepper flakes, salt, and pepper.

5. Add cooked spaghetti to the skillet and toss to combine with the shrimp and sauce.

6. Serve lemon garlic shrimp pasta hot, garnished with chopped fresh parsley.

12. Sweet Potato and Black Bean Enchiladas:

- *Ingredients:*

- 2 medium sweet potatoes, peeled and diced

- 1 tablespoon olive oil

- 1/2 teaspoon chili powder

- 1/2 teaspoon cumin

- 1 can (15 oz) black beans, drained and rinsed

- 1 cup diced tomatoes

- 1 cup shredded Monterey Jack cheese

- 8 whole wheat tortillas

- Enchilada sauce for topping

- Chopped fresh cilantro for garnish

- ### Instructions:

1. Preheat oven to 375°F (190°C). Grease a baking dish with olive oil.

2. Toss diced sweet potatoes with olive oil, chili powder, and cumin. Spread sweet potatoes on a baking sheet and roast for 20-25 minutes, or until tender.

3. In a large bowl, mash half of the roasted sweet potatoes. Add black beans, diced tomatoes, and shredded Monterey Jack cheese to the bowl. Stir to combine.

4. Place a spoonful of the sweet potato and black bean mixture onto each whole wheat tortilla. Roll up the tortillas and place them seam-side down in the prepared baking dish.

5. Pour enchilada sauce over the rolled tortillas, covering them completely.

6. Bake enchiladas for 20-25 minutes, or until heated through and cheese is melted.

7. Garnish with chopped fresh cilantro before serving.

13. Broccoli and Mushroom Stir-Fry:

- ### Ingredients:

  - 2 tablespoons olive oil

  - 2 cloves garlic, minced

  - 1 teaspoon grated ginger

  - 2 cups broccoli florets

  - 2 cups sliced mushrooms

- 1 red bell pepper, sliced

- 1/4 cup soy sauce

- 1 tablespoon honey

- Cooked brown rice for serving

- Sesame seeds for garnish

- ### *Instructions:*

1. Heat olive oil in a large skillet or wok over medium-high heat. Add minced garlic and grated ginger, and cook for 1 minute.

2. Add broccoli florets, sliced mushrooms, and sliced red bell pepper to the skillet. Stir-fry until vegetables are tender-crisp.

3. In a small bowl, whisk together soy sauce and honey. Pour the sauce over the vegetables and toss to coat evenly.

4. Serve broccoli and mushroom stir-fry over cooked brown rice.

5. Garnish with sesame seeds before serving.

14. Baked Eggplant Parmesan:

- ### *Ingredients:*

  - 2 medium eggplants, sliced into rounds

  - 2 eggs, beaten

  - 1 cup whole wheat breadcrumbs

  - 1/4 cup grated Parmesan cheese

  - 2 cups marinara sauce

  - 1 cup shredded mozzarella cheese

  - Chopped fresh basil for garnish

- *Instructions:*

    1. Preheat oven to 400°F (200°C). Line a baking sheet with parchment paper.

    2. Dip eggplant slices into beaten eggs, then coat with whole wheat breadcrumbs mixed with grated Parmesan cheese.

    3. Place coated eggplant slices on the prepared baking sheet. Bake for 15-20 minutes, or until golden brown and crispy.

    4. Spread marinara sauce in the bottom of a baking dish. Arrange baked eggplant slices on top of the sauce.

    5. Top eggplant slices with shredded mozzarella cheese.

    6. Bake eggplant Parmesan for an additional 10-15 minutes, or until cheese is melted and bubbly.

    7. Garnish with chopped fresh basil before serving.

15. Lemon Herb Roasted Chicken and Vegetables:

- *Ingredients:*

    - 4 bone-in, skin-on chicken thighs

    - 2 tablespoons olive oil

    - Zest and juice of 1 lemon

    - 2 cloves garlic, minced

    - 1 teaspoon dried thyme

    - 1 teaspoon dried rosemary

    - 2 cups mixed vegetables (such as carrots, potatoes, and Brussels sprouts), chopped

    - Salt and pepper to taste

- *Instructions:*

    1. Preheat oven to 400°F (200°C). Line a baking sheet with parchment paper.

    2. In a bowl, whisk together olive oil, lemon zest, lemon juice, minced garlic, dried thyme, and dried rosemary.

    3. Place chicken thighs on the prepared baking sheet. Arrange mixed vegetables around the chicken.

    4. Brush chicken thighs and vegetables with the lemon herb mixture. Season with salt and pepper.

    5. Roast chicken and vegetables in the preheated oven for 35-40 minutes, or until chicken is cooked through and vegetables are tender.

    6. Serve hot, with a side of whole grain bread or salad.

These recipes offer a variety of nutritious and flavorful options for cancer-friendly dinners. Enjoy experimenting with different ingredients and flavors!

16. *Salmon and Asparagus Foil Packets:*

- *Ingredients:*

    - 2 salmon fillets

    - 1 bunch asparagus, trimmed

    - 2 tablespoons olive oil

    - 2 cloves garlic, minced

    - Zest and juice of 1 lemon

    - Salt and pepper to taste

    - Fresh dill for garnish

- *Instructions:*

1. Preheat oven to 400°F (200°C). Cut two large pieces of aluminum foil.

2. Place a salmon fillet on each piece of foil. Arrange asparagus around the salmon.

3. In a small bowl, whisk together olive oil, minced garlic, lemon zest, and lemon juice. Drizzle over the salmon and asparagus. Season with salt and pepper.

4. Fold the foil over the salmon and asparagus to create packets, sealing tightly.

5. Place foil packets on a baking sheet and bake for 15-20 minutes, or until salmon is cooked through and flakes easily with a fork.

6. Garnish with fresh dill before serving.

17. Quinoa Stuffed Bell Peppers:

- ### Ingredients:

  - 4 bell peppers, halved and seeds removed

  - 1 cup cooked quinoa

  - 1 can (15 oz) black beans, drained and rinsed

  - 1 cup corn kernels

  - 1 cup diced tomatoes

  - 1 teaspoon chili powder

  - 1/2 teaspoon cumin

  - 1/2 cup shredded cheddar cheese

  - Chopped fresh cilantro for garnish

- ### Instructions:

1. Preheat oven to 375°F (190°C). Grease a baking dish with olive oil.

2. In a large bowl, combine cooked quinoa, black beans, corn kernels, diced tomatoes, chili powder, and cumin.

3.	Spoon quinoa mixture into halved bell peppers, pressing down gently to pack the filling.

4.	Place stuffed bell peppers in the prepared baking dish. Cover with foil and bake for 25-30 minutes.

5.	Remove foil, sprinkle shredded cheddar cheese over the stuffed peppers, and bake for an additional 5 minutes, or until cheese is melted and bubbly.

6.	Garnish with chopped fresh cilantro before serving.

## 18.	Vegetable Lentil Soup:

- ### Ingredients:

  - 1 tablespoon olive oil

  - 1 onion, diced

  - 2 carrots, diced

  - 2 stalks celery, diced

  - 2 cloves garlic, minced

  - 1 cup dried green lentils

  - 6 cups vegetable broth

  - 1 can (15 oz) diced tomatoes

  - 1 teaspoon dried thyme

  - 1 teaspoon dried oregano

  - Salt and pepper to taste

  - Chopped fresh parsley for garnish

- ### Instructions:

1.	Heat olive oil in a large pot over medium heat. Add diced onion, carrots, celery, and minced garlic. Cook until vegetables are softened.

2.   Add dried green lentils, vegetable broth, diced tomatoes, dried thyme, and dried oregano to the pot. Bring to a boil, then reduce heat and simmer for 20-25 minutes, or until lentils are tender.

3.   Season with salt and pepper to taste.

4.   Serve vegetable lentil soup hot, garnished with chopped fresh parsley.

19.   *Mediterranean Chickpea Salad:*

- *Ingredients:*

  - 1 can (15 oz) chickpeas, drained and rinsed

  - 1 cucumber, diced

  - 1 cup cherry tomatoes, halved

  - 1/2 red onion, thinly sliced

  - 1/4 cup Kalamata olives, pitted and halved

  - 1/4 cup crumbled feta cheese

  - 2 tablespoons chopped fresh parsley

  - 2 tablespoons extra virgin olive oil

  - 1 tablespoon lemon juice

  - 1 teaspoon dried oregano

  - Salt and pepper to taste

- *Instructions:*

1.   In a large bowl, combine chickpeas, diced cucumber, cherry tomatoes, sliced red onion, Kalamata olives, crumbled feta cheese, and chopped fresh parsley.

2.   In a small bowl, whisk together extra virgin olive oil, lemon juice, dried oregano, salt, and pepper.

3.   Pour the dressing over the chickpea salad and toss to combine.

4.   Serve Mediterranean chickpea salad chilled or at room temperature.

20. *Turkey and Vegetable Meatballs:*

- *Ingredients:*

  - 1 lb ground turkey

  - 1/2 cup grated zucchini

  - 1/2 cup grated carrot

  - 1/4 cup finely chopped onion

  - 2 cloves garlic, minced

  - 1/4 cup whole wheat breadcrumbs

  - 1 egg

  - 2 tablespoons chopped fresh parsley

  - 1 teaspoon dried oregano

  - 1/2 teaspoon salt

  - 1/4 teaspoon black pepper

  - Olive oil for cooking

- *Instructions:*

1.   Preheat oven to 400°F (200°C). Line a baking sheet with parchment paper.

2.   In a large bowl, combine ground turkey, grated zucchini, grated carrot, chopped onion, minced garlic, whole wheat breadcrumbs, egg, chopped fresh parsley, dried oregano, salt, and black pepper. Mix until well combined.

3.   Shape the turkey mixture into meatballs and place them on the prepared baking sheet.

4.   Bake meatballs in the preheated oven for 20-25 minutes, or until cooked through and browned.

5.   Serve turkey and vegetable meatballs hot, with your favorite marinara sauce or over whole wheat pasta.

21.   *Sesame Ginger Tofu Stir-Fry:*

- ### *Ingredients:*

  - 1 block (14 oz) extra firm tofu, pressed and cubed

  - 2 tablespoons soy sauce

  - 1 tablespoon sesame oil

  - 1 tablespoon rice vinegar

  - 1 tablespoon honey or maple syrup

  - 2 cloves garlic, minced

  - 1 tablespoon minced ginger

  - 2 cups mixed vegetables (such as bell peppers, broccoli, and snap peas)

  - Cooked brown rice for serving

  - Sesame seeds and sliced green onions for garnish

- ### *Instructions:*

1.   In a bowl, whisk together soy sauce, sesame oil, rice vinegar, honey or maple syrup, minced garlic, and minced ginger.

2.   Heat a large skillet or wok over medium-high heat. Add cubed tofu and cook until golden brown on all sides.

3.   Remove tofu from the skillet and set aside. Add mixed vegetables to the skillet and stir-fry until crisp-tender.

4.   Return tofu to the skillet and pour the sauce over the tofu and vegetables. Cook for an additional 2-3 minutes, or until heated through.

5. Serve sesame ginger tofu stir-fry hot, over cooked brown rice. Garnish with sesame seeds and sliced green onions.

22. Vegetarian Chili:

- **Ingredients:**

    - 1 tablespoon olive oil

    - 1 onion, diced

    - 2 cloves garlic, minced

    - 1 bell pepper, diced

    - 1 jalapeno pepper, seeded and diced

    - 1 zucchini, diced

    - 1 cup corn kernels

    - 1 can (15 oz) black beans, drained and rinsed

    - 1 can (15 oz) kidney beans, drained and rinsed

    - 1 can (15 oz) diced tomatoes

    - 2 cups vegetable broth

    - 2 tablespoons chili powder

    - 1 teaspoon ground cumin

    - 1/2 teaspoon smoked paprika

    - Salt and pepper to taste

    - Chopped fresh cilantro for garnish

- **Instructions:**

1. Heat olive oil in a large pot over medium heat. Add diced onion, minced garlic, diced bell pepper, and diced jalapeno pepper. Cook until vegetables are softened.

2. Add diced zucchini, corn kernels, black beans, kidney beans, diced tomatoes, vegetable broth, chili powder, ground cumin, and smoked paprika to the pot. Stir to combine.

3. Bring the chili to a simmer and cook for 20-25 minutes, stirring occasionally.

4. Season with salt and pepper to taste.

5. Serve vegetarian chili hot, garnished with chopped fresh cilantro.

23. Baked Pesto Salmon:

- ### Ingredients:

  - 2 salmon fillets

  - 2 tablespoons prepared pesto

  - 1 tablespoon lemon juice

  - 1 tablespoon olive oil

  - Salt and pepper to taste

  - Lemon slices for garnish

  - Fresh basil for garnish

- ### Instructions:

1. Preheat oven to 400°F (200°C). Line a baking sheet with parchment paper.

2. Place salmon fillets on the prepared baking sheet. Spread prepared pesto over the top of each fillet.

3. Drizzle lemon juice and olive oil over the salmon. Season with salt and pepper.

4. Bake salmon in the preheated oven for 12-15 minutes, or until salmon is cooked through and flakes easily with a fork.

5. Garnish with lemon slices and fresh basil before serving.

24. Spinach and Mushroom Quiche:

- Ingredients:
  - 1 pie crust (store-bought or homemade)
  - 1 tablespoon olive oil
  - 1 onion, diced
  - 2 cups sliced mushrooms
  - 2 cups fresh baby spinach
  - 4 large eggs
  - 1 cup milk (any type)
  - 1/2 cup shredded cheddar cheese
  - Salt and pepper to taste
  - Pinch of nutmeg

- ***Instructions:***

1. Preheat oven to 375°F (190°C). Place pie crust in a pie dish and crimp the edges.

2. In a skillet, heat olive oil over medium heat. Add diced onion and sliced mushrooms. Cook until mushrooms are golden brown and onions are softened.

3. Add fresh baby spinach to the skillet and cook until wilted. Remove from heat and let cool slightly.

4. In a bowl, whisk together eggs, milk, shredded cheddar cheese, salt, pepper, and a pinch of nutmeg.

5. Spread the mushroom, spinach, and onion mixture evenly over the bottom of the pie crust. Pour the egg mixture over the vegetables.

6. Bake quiche in the preheated oven for 35-40 minutes, or until set and golden brown.

7. Let quiche cool for a few minutes before slicing and serving.

25. Lemon Garlic Shrimp Pasta:

- **Ingredients:**

  - 8 oz whole wheat spaghetti

  - 1 tablespoon olive oil

  - 1 lb shrimp, peeled and deveined

  - 4 cloves garlic, minced

  - Zest and juice of 1 lemon

  - 1/4 cup chopped fresh parsley

  - Salt and pepper to taste

  - Grated Parmesan cheese for serving

- **Instructions:**

1. Cook whole wheat spaghetti according to package instructions until al dente. Drain and set aside.

2. In a large skillet, heat olive oil over medium heat. Add peeled and deveined shrimp and minced garlic. Cook until shrimp are pink and opaque.

3. Add cooked spaghetti to the skillet. Toss with lemon zest, lemon juice, chopped fresh parsley, salt, and pepper.

4. Serve lemon garlic shrimp pasta hot, garnished with grated Parmesan cheese.

26. Butternut Squash and Lentil Curry:

- **Ingredients:**

  - 1 tablespoon coconut oil

  - 1 onion, diced

  - 2 cloves garlic, minced

- 1 tablespoon grated ginger

- 2 cups diced butternut squash

- 1 cup dried green lentils

- 1 can (14 oz) coconut milk

- 2 cups vegetable broth

- 2 tablespoons red curry paste

- 1 tablespoon curry powder

- 1 teaspoon ground turmeric

- Salt and pepper to taste

- Chopped fresh cilantro for garnish

- *Instructions:*

1. In a large pot, heat coconut oil over medium heat. Add diced onion, minced garlic, and grated ginger. Cook until onions are translucent.

2. Add diced butternut squash, dried green lentils, coconut milk, vegetable broth, red curry paste, curry powder, and ground turmeric to the pot. Stir to combine.

3. Bring the curry to a boil, then reduce heat and simmer for 20-25 minutes, or until butternut squash and lentils are tender.

4. Season with salt and pepper to taste.

5. Serve butternut squash and lentil curry hot, garnished with chopped fresh cilantro.

27. Caprese Stuffed Portobello Mushrooms:

- *Ingredients:*

- 4 large portobello mushrooms

- 2 tablespoons balsamic vinegar

- 2 tablespoons olive oil

- 2 cloves garlic, minced

- 1 cup cherry tomatoes, halved

- 4 oz fresh mozzarella cheese, sliced

- 1/4 cup chopped fresh basil

- Salt and pepper to taste

- *Instructions:*

1. Preheat oven to 400°F (200°C). Remove stems from portobello mushrooms and gently scrape out the gills.

2. In a small bowl, whisk together balsamic vinegar, olive oil, and minced garlic.

3. Brush the inside of each portobello mushroom with the balsamic mixture. Place mushrooms on a baking sheet, gill side up.

4. Fill each mushroom with halved cherry tomatoes, sliced fresh mozzarella cheese, and chopped fresh basil. Season with salt and pepper.

5. Bake stuffed portobello mushrooms in the preheated oven for 15-20 minutes, or until mushrooms are tender and cheese is melted and bubbly.

6. Serve caprese stuffed portobello mushrooms hot, garnished with additional chopped fresh basil.

28. Honey Garlic Tofu Stir-Fry:

- *Ingredients:*

  - 1 block (14 oz) extra firm tofu, pressed and cubed

  - 2 tablespoons soy sauce

  - 1 tablespoon honey

  - 2 cloves garlic, minced

- 1 tablespoon sesame oil

- 1 tablespoon cornstarch

- 2 tablespoons water

- 2 cups mixed vegetables (such as bell peppers, broccoli, and snap peas)

- Cooked brown rice for serving

- Sliced green onions for garnish

- *Instructions:*

1. In a bowl, whisk together soy sauce, honey, minced garlic, sesame oil, cornstarch, and water.

2. Heat a large skillet or wok over medium-high heat. Add cubed tofu and cook until golden brown on all sides.

3. Remove tofu from the skillet and set aside. Add mixed vegetables to the skillet and stir-fry until crisp-tender.

4. Return tofu to the skillet and pour the sauce over the tofu and vegetables. Cook for an additional 2-3 minutes, or until heated through and sauce has thickened.

5. Serve honey garlic tofu stir-fry hot, over cooked brown rice. Garnish with sliced green onions.

29. Eggplant Parmesan:

- *Ingredients:*

  - 1 large eggplant, sliced into rounds

  - Salt

  - 1 cup whole wheat breadcrumbs

  - 1/2 cup grated Parmesan cheese

  - 2 eggs, beaten

  - 2 cups marinara sauce

- 1 cup shredded mozzarella cheese

- Fresh basil leaves for garnish

- ### *Instructions:*

1. Place eggplant slices in a colander and sprinkle with salt. Let sit for 30 minutes to draw out moisture. Pat dry with paper towels.

2. Preheat oven to 375°F (190°C). Line a baking sheet with parchment paper.

3. In a shallow dish, combine whole wheat breadcrumbs and grated Parmesan cheese. Dip eggplant slices in beaten eggs, then coat with breadcrumb mixture.

4. Place breaded eggplant slices on the prepared baking sheet. Bake in the preheated oven for 20-25 minutes, or until golden brown and crispy.

5. Spread marinara sauce in the bottom of a baking dish. Arrange baked eggplant slices over the sauce. Top with remaining marinara sauce and shredded mozzarella cheese.

6. Bake eggplant Parmesan for an additional 15-20 minutes, or until cheese is melted and bubbly.

7. Garnish with fresh basil leaves before serving.

30. *Miso Glazed Salmon:*

- ### *Ingredients:*

  - 2 salmon fillets

  - 2 tablespoons white miso paste

  - 1 tablespoon honey

  - 1 tablespoon soy sauce

  - 1 tablespoon rice vinegar

  - 1 teaspoon grated ginger

  - 1 clove garlic, minced

- Sesame seeds for garnish

- Sliced green onions for garnish

- *Instructions:*

1. Preheat broiler to high. Line a baking sheet with foil and lightly grease with olive oil.

2. In a small bowl, whisk together white miso paste, honey, soy sauce, rice vinegar, grated ginger, and minced garlic.

3. Place salmon fillets on the prepared baking sheet. Brush the miso glaze over the salmon.

4. Broil salmon for 8-10 minutes, or until salmon is cooked through and caramelized on top.

5. Garnish miso glazed salmon with sesame seeds and sliced green onions before serving.

31. Quinoa Stuffed Acorn Squash:

- *Ingredients:*

  - 2 acorn squash, halved and seeds removed

  - 1 cup cooked quinoa

  - 1/2 cup dried cranberries

  - 1/2 cup chopped pecans

  - 2 tablespoons maple syrup

  - 1 teaspoon ground cinnamon

  - Salt and pepper to taste

- *Instructions:*

1. Preheat oven to 400°F (200°C). Place acorn squash halves cut side down on a baking sheet lined with parchment paper. Bake for 30 minutes.

2. In a bowl, combine cooked quinoa, dried cranberries, chopped pecans, maple syrup, ground cinnamon, salt, and pepper.

3. Remove acorn squash from the oven and flip over. Fill each squash half with the quinoa mixture.

4. Return stuffed acorn squash to the oven and bake for an additional 15 minutes.

5. Serve quinoa stuffed acorn squash hot, as a nutritious and flavorful dinner option.

These dinner recipes offer a variety of nutritious options for those looking to maintain a healthy lifestyle while also enjoying delicious and satisfying meals.

CHAPTER 5: STAPLE CARBOHYDRATES

Staple carbohydrates are primary sources of energy in the diet and typically form the basis of many meals. They include foods like whole grains, rice, pasta, bread, and starchy vegetables like potatoes. These foods are considered cancer-friendly for several reasons:

1. **High in Fiber:** Whole grains and starchy vegetables are rich in dietary fiber, which promotes healthy digestion, helps maintain bowel regularity, and may reduce the risk of certain types of cancer, particularly colorectal cancer. Fiber also helps control blood sugar levels and contributes to a feeling of fullness, which can aid in weight management.

2. **Nutrient-Rich:** Staple carbohydrates are often rich in essential nutrients such as vitamins, minerals, and antioxidants. For example, whole grains contain B vitamins, iron, magnesium, and selenium, while starchy vegetables like sweet potatoes provide beta-carotene, vitamin C, and potassium. These nutrients play various roles in supporting overall health and immune function, which may help protect against cancer development.

3. **Low Glycemic Index:** Whole grains and certain starchy vegetables have a low glycemic index (GI), meaning they cause a slower and steadier increase in blood sugar levels compared to refined carbohydrates. Diets rich in low-GI foods have been associated with a reduced risk of certain cancers, as high blood sugar and insulin levels may promote cancer cell growth.

4. **Antioxidant Properties:** Many staple carbohydrates contain antioxidants that help neutralize harmful free radicals and protect cells from damage. For example, whole grains contain phenolic compounds.

1. Quinoa Salad with Chickpeas and Vegetables:

- *Ingredients:*

    - 1 cup quinoa, rinsed

    - 2 cups water or vegetable broth

- 1 can (15 oz) chickpeas, drained and rinsed

- 1 cucumber, diced

- 1 bell pepper, diced

- 1/4 cup chopped fresh parsley

- 1/4 cup chopped fresh mint

- Juice of 1 lemon

- 2 tablespoons olive oil

- Salt and pepper to taste

- *Instructions:*

1. In a saucepan, bring the quinoa and water or broth to a boil. Reduce heat, cover, and simmer for 15-20 minutes, or until quinoa is cooked and liquid is absorbed. Fluff with a fork and let cool.

2. In a large bowl, combine cooked quinoa, chickpeas, diced cucumber, diced bell pepper, chopped parsley, and chopped mint.

3. In a small bowl, whisk together lemon juice, olive oil, salt, and pepper. Pour over the quinoa mixture and toss to combine.

4. Serve quinoa salad chilled or at room temperature.

2. Brown Rice Stir-Fry with Tofu and Vegetables:

- *Ingredients:*

  - 1 cup brown rice

  - 2 cups water

  - 1 tablespoon sesame oil

  - 1 block (14 oz) firm tofu, cubed

  - 2 cups mixed vegetables (broccoli, bell peppers, carrots, snap peas)

- 2 cloves garlic, minced

- 2 tablespoons soy sauce

- 1 tablespoon rice vinegar

- 1 teaspoon grated ginger

- Sesame seeds for garnish

- Sliced green onions for garnish

- *Instructions:*

1. In a saucepan, combine brown rice and water. Bring to a boil, then reduce heat, cover, and simmer for 45-50 minutes, or until rice is tender and water is absorbed.

2. In a large skillet or wok, heat sesame oil over medium-high heat. Add cubed tofu and cook until golden brown on all sides. Remove tofu from skillet and set aside.

3. In the same skillet, add mixed vegetables and minced garlic. Stir-fry until vegetables are tender-crisp.

4. Return tofu to the skillet. Add cooked brown rice, soy sauce, rice vinegar, and grated ginger. Stir-fry until everything is heated through and well combined.

5. Garnish with sesame seeds and sliced green onions before serving.

3. Barley and Vegetable Soup:

- *Ingredients:*

  - 1 cup pearl barley

  - 6 cups vegetable broth

  - 2 carrots, diced

  - 2 celery stalks, diced

  - 1 onion, diced

- 2 cloves garlic, minced

- 1 can (15 oz) diced tomatoes

- 2 cups chopped kale or spinach

- 1 teaspoon dried thyme

- Salt and pepper to taste

- Fresh parsley for garnish

- **Instructions:**

  1. In a large pot, combine pearl barley and vegetable broth. Bring to a boil, then reduce heat and simmer for 30-35 minutes, or until barley is tender.

  2. Add diced carrots, diced celery, diced onion, minced garlic, diced tomatoes (with juices), chopped kale or spinach, dried thyme, salt, and pepper to the pot.

  3. Continue to simmer for an additional 15-20 minutes, or until vegetables are tender.

  4. Adjust seasoning if needed and serve hot, garnished with fresh parsley.

4. Millet Pilaf with Roasted Vegetables:

- **Ingredients:**

  - 1 cup millet

  - 2 cups vegetable broth

  - 1 sweet potato, peeled and diced

  - 2 carrots, peeled and diced

  - 1 red onion, diced

  - 1 bell pepper, diced

  - 2 tablespoons olive oil

- 1 teaspoon dried thyme

- Salt and pepper to taste

- Fresh parsley for garnish

- ***Instructions:***

1. Preheat oven to 400°F (200°C). Line a baking sheet with parchment paper.

2. In a pot, bring vegetable broth to a boil. Add millet, cover, and simmer for 20-25 minutes, or until millet is cooked and liquid is absorbed. Fluff with a fork and let cool.

3. Place diced sweet potato, diced carrots, diced red onion, and diced bell pepper on the prepared baking sheet. Drizzle with olive oil, sprinkle with dried thyme, salt, and pepper. Toss to coat.

4. Roast vegetables in the preheated oven for 25-30 minutes, or until tender and slightly caramelized.

5. In a large bowl, combine cooked millet and roasted vegetables. Toss gently to combine.

6. Serve millet pilaf warm, garnished with fresh parsley.

5. Lentil and Brown Rice Casserole:

- ***Ingredients:***

- 1 cup brown rice

- 1/2 cup green lentils

- 3 cups vegetable broth

- 1 onion, diced

- 2 cloves garlic, minced

- 1 bell pepper, diced

- 1 can (15 oz) diced tomatoes

- 1 teaspoon dried oregano

- 1 teaspoon dried basil

- Salt and pepper to taste

- 1/2 cup grated Parmesan cheese (optional)

- *Instructions:*

1. Preheat oven to 375°F (190°C). Lightly grease a baking dish.

2. In a large bowl, combine brown rice, green lentils, diced onion, minced garlic, diced bell pepper, diced tomatoes (with juices), dried oregano, dried basil, salt, and pepper.

3. Pour the mixture into the prepared baking dish. Spread it out evenly.

4. Pour vegetable broth over the rice and lentil mixture.

5. Cover the baking dish with foil and bake in the preheated oven for 45-50 minutes, or until rice and lentils are tender and most of the liquid is absorbed.

6. If desired, sprinkle grated Parmesan cheese over the casserole during the last 10 minutes of baking.

7. Let cool slightly before serving.

6. Wild Rice Salad with Cranberries and Almonds:

- *Ingredients:*

  - 1 cup wild rice

  - 3 cups water or vegetable broth

  - 1/2 cup dried cranberries

  - 1/4 cup sliced almonds, toasted

- 2 green onions, thinly sliced

- 2 tablespoons chopped fresh parsley

- Juice of 1 lemon

- 2 tablespoons olive oil

- Salt and pepper to taste

- *Instructions:*

1. In a saucepan, bring the wild rice and water or broth to a boil. Reduce heat, cover, and simmer for 45-50 minutes, or until rice is tender and water is absorbed. Fluff with a fork and let cool.

2. In a large bowl, combine cooked wild rice, dried cranberries, toasted sliced almonds, thinly sliced green onions, and chopped fresh parsley.

3. In a small bowl, whisk together lemon juice, olive oil, salt, and pepper. Pour over the rice mixture and toss to combine.

4. Serve wild rice salad chilled or at room temperature.

7. Bulgur and Chickpea Salad:

- *Ingredients:*

  - 1 cup bulgur wheat

  - 2 cups water or vegetable broth

  - 1 can (15 oz) chickpeas, drained and rinsed

  - 1 cucumber, diced

  - 1 tomato, diced

  - 1/4 cup chopped fresh mint

  - 1/4 cup chopped fresh parsley

- Juice of 1 lemon

- 2 tablespoons olive oil

- Salt and pepper to taste

- **_Instructions:_**

  1. In a saucepan, bring bulgur wheat and water or broth to a boil. Reduce heat, cover, and simmer for 12-15 minutes, or until bulgur is tender and liquid is absorbed. Fluff with a fork and let cool.

  2. In a large bowl, combine cooked bulgur, chickpeas, diced cucumber, diced tomato, chopped fresh mint, and chopped fresh parsley.

  3. In a small bowl, whisk together lemon juice, olive oil, salt, and pepper. Pour over the bulgur mixture and toss to combine.

  4. Serve bulgur and chickpea salad chilled or at room temperature.

8. Spelt Pasta with Roasted Vegetables and Pesto:

- **_Ingredients:_**

  - 8 oz spelt pasta

  - 1 eggplant, diced

  - 1 zucchini, diced

  - 1 red bell pepper, diced

  - 1 yellow bell pepper, diced

  - 2 tablespoons olive oil

  - Salt and pepper to taste

  - 1/4 cup prepared pesto

  - Grated Parmesan cheese for serving (optional)

- *Instructions:*

1. Preheat oven to 400°F (200°C). Line a baking sheet with parchment paper.

2. Place diced eggplant, diced zucchini, diced red bell pepper, and diced yellow bell pepper on the prepared baking sheet. Drizzle with olive oil, season with salt and pepper, and toss to coat.

3. Roast vegetables in the preheated oven for 20-25 minutes, or until tender and slightly caramelized.

4. While the vegetables are roasting, cook spelt pasta according to package instructions. Drain and set aside.

5. In a large bowl, toss cooked spelt pasta with roasted vegetables and prepared pesto until well combined.

6. Serve spelt pasta with roasted vegetables hot, garnished with grated Parmesan cheese if desired.

9. Sorghum Salad with Pomegranate and Feta:

- *Ingredients:*

  - 1 cup sorghum

  - 3 cups water or vegetable broth

  - Seeds from 1 pomegranate

  - 1/4 cup crumbled feta cheese

  - 1/4 cup chopped fresh mint

  - 1/4 cup chopped fresh parsley

  - Juice of 1 lemon

  - 2 tablespoons olive oil

  - Salt and pepper to taste

- *Instructions:*

  1. In a saucepan, bring sorghum and water or broth to a boil. Reduce heat, cover, and simmer for 50-60 minutes, or until sorghum is tender and liquid is absorbed. Fluff with a fork and let cool.

  2. In a large bowl, combine cooked sorghum, pomegranate seeds, crumbled feta cheese, chopped fresh mint, and chopped fresh parsley.

  3. In a small bowl, whisk together lemon juice, olive oil, salt, and pepper. Pour over the sorghum mixture and toss to combine.

  4. Serve sorghum salad chilled or at room temperature.

10. Black Rice Stir-Fry with Tofu and Vegetables:

- *Ingredients:*

  - 1 cup black rice
  - 2 cups water
  - 1 tablespoon sesame oil
  - 1 block (14 oz) firm tofu, cubed
  - 2 cups mixed vegetables (broccoli, bell peppers, carrots, snap peas)
  - 2 cloves garlic, minced
  - 2 tablespoons soy sauce
  - 1 tablespoon rice vinegar
  - 1 teaspoon grated ginger
  - Sesame seeds for garnish
  - Sliced green onions for garnish

- *Instructions:*

1. In a saucepan, combine black rice and water. Bring to a boil, then reduce heat, cover, and simmer for 30-35 minutes, or until rice is tender and water is absorbed.

2. In a large skillet or wok, heat sesame oil over medium-high heat. Add cubed tofu and cook until golden brown on all sides. Remove tofu from skillet and set aside.

3. In the same skillet, add mixed vegetables and minced garlic. Stir-fry until vegetables are tender-crisp.

4. Return tofu to the skillet. Add cooked black rice, soy sauce, rice vinegar, and grated ginger. Stir-fry until everything is heated through and well combined.

5. Garnish with sesame seeds and sliced green onions before serving.

11. *Sesame Ginger Buckwheat Noodles:*

- ***Ingredients:***

  - 8 oz buckwheat noodles

  - 2 tablespoons sesame oil

  - 2 tablespoons soy sauce

  - 1 tablespoon rice vinegar

  - 1 tablespoon honey or maple syrup

  - 1 teaspoon grated ginger

  - 2 cloves garlic, minced

  - 1/4 cup chopped green onions

  - 1/4 cup shredded carrots

  - Toasted sesame seeds for garnish

- ***Instructions:***

1. Cook buckwheat noodles according to package instructions. Drain and rinse under cold water.

2. In a small bowl, whisk together sesame oil, soy sauce, rice vinegar, honey or maple syrup, grated ginger, and minced garlic to make the dressing.

3. In a large bowl, toss cooked buckwheat noodles with chopped green onions and shredded carrots.

4. Pour the dressing over the noodles and vegetables. Toss until well coated.

5. Serve sesame ginger buckwheat noodles garnished with toasted sesame seeds.

12. Red Lentil Curry with Brown Rice:

- ### Ingredients:

  - 1 cup brown rice

  - 2 cups water

  - 1 cup red lentils, rinsed

  - 1 onion, diced

  - 2 cloves garlic, minced

  - 1 tablespoon grated ginger

  - 1 can (14 oz) coconut milk

  - 1 can (14 oz) diced tomatoes

  - 2 tablespoons curry powder

  - 1 teaspoon ground turmeric

  - Salt and pepper to taste

  - Fresh cilantro for garnish

- ### Instructions:

1. In a saucepan, combine brown rice and water. Bring to a boil, then reduce heat, cover, and simmer for 45-50 minutes, or until rice is tender and water is absorbed.

2. In a separate large pot, heat a little oil over medium heat. Add diced onion, minced garlic, and grated ginger. Cook until softened and fragrant.

3. Stir in curry powder and ground turmeric, and cook for another minute.

4. Add red lentils, coconut milk, diced tomatoes (with juices), salt, and pepper to the pot. Bring to a simmer and cook for 20-25 minutes, or until lentils are tender and curry has thickened.

5. Serve red lentil curry over cooked brown rice, garnished with fresh cilantro.

13. Cauliflower Fried Rice:

- ### Ingredients:

  - 1 small head cauliflower, riced (about 4 cups)

  - 2 tablespoons sesame oil

  - 2 eggs, lightly beaten

  - 1 cup mixed vegetables (peas, carrots, corn)

  - 2 cloves garlic, minced

  - 2 tablespoons soy sauce

  - 1 tablespoon rice vinegar

  - 1 teaspoon grated ginger

  - 2 green onions, sliced

  - Sesame seeds for garnish

- ### Instructions:

1. Heat 1 tablespoon of sesame oil in a large skillet or wok over medium heat. Add beaten eggs and scramble until cooked through. Remove from skillet and set aside.

2. Add the remaining tablespoon of sesame oil to the skillet. Add minced garlic and grated ginger, and cook until fragrant.

3. Add riced cauliflower and mixed vegetables to the skillet. Cook, stirring frequently, until vegetables are tender-crisp.

4. Return scrambled eggs to the skillet. Stir in soy sauce and rice vinegar, and cook for an additional 2-3 minutes.

5. Garnish cauliflower fried rice with sliced green onions and sesame seeds before serving.

14. Barley Risotto with Mushrooms and Spinach:

- **Ingredients:**

  - 1 cup pearl barley

  - 4 cups vegetable broth

  - 2 tablespoons olive oil

  - 1 onion, diced

  - 2 cloves garlic, minced

  - 8 oz mushrooms, sliced

  - 2 cups baby spinach

  - 1/4 cup grated Parmesan cheese

  - Salt and pepper to taste

  - Chopped fresh parsley for garnish

- **Instructions:**

1. In a saucepan, bring vegetable broth to a simmer and keep it warm over low heat.

2. In a separate large pot, heat olive oil over medium heat. Add diced onion and minced garlic, and cook until softened.

3. Add sliced mushrooms to the pot and cook until they release their juices and start to brown.

4. Stir in pearl barley and cook for 1-2 minutes, stirring constantly.

5. Begin adding the warm vegetable broth to the pot, one ladleful at a time, stirring frequently and allowing the barley to absorb the liquid before adding more. Continue this process until the barley is tender and creamy, about 30-40 minutes.

6. Stir in baby spinach and grated Parmesan cheese until spinach wilts and cheese is melted. Season with salt and pepper to taste.

7. Serve barley risotto hot, garnished with chopped fresh parsley.

15. Sesame Quinoa Bowl with Tofu and Vegetables:

- **Ingredients:**

  - 1 cup quinoa, rinsed

  - 2 cups vegetable broth

  - 1 block (14 oz) firm tofu, cubed

  - 2 tablespoons soy sauce

  - 1 tablespoon sesame oil

  - 2 tablespoons olive oil

  - 2 cups mixed vegetables (bell peppers, broccoli, snap peas)

  - 2 cloves garlic, minced

  - 2 tablespoons sesame seeds

- Sliced green onions for garnish

- ### *Instructions:*

  1. In a saucepan, bring quinoa and vegetable broth to a boil. Reduce heat, cover, and simmer for 15-20 minutes, or until quinoa is cooked and liquid is absorbed. Fluff with a fork and let cool.

  2. In a large skillet or wok, heat olive oil over medium-high heat. Add cubed tofu and cook until golden brown on all sides. Remove tofu from skillet and set aside.

  3. In the same skillet, add minced garlic and mixed vegetables. Stir-fry until vegetables are tender-crisp.

  4. Return tofu to the skillet. Add cooked quinoa, soy sauce, and sesame oil. Stir-fry until everything is heated through and well combined.

  5. Sprinkle sesame seeds and sliced green onions over the quinoa bowl before serving.

These recipes provide a variety of delicious and nutritious options featuring grains and rice, perfect for individuals seeking cancer-friendly meal ideas. Enjoy exploring these wholesome dishes!

CHAPTER 6: PULSES

Pulses are the edible seeds of plants in the legume family. They are harvested dry and include various types of beans, lentils, and peas. Pulses are a rich source of protein, fiber, vitamins, and minerals, making them an essential part of a healthy diet. They are often used in cooking to create nutritious and delicious dishes, ranging from soups and stews to salads and side dishes. Pulses are also known for their sustainability and environmental benefits, as they enrich the soil with nitrogen and require less water to grow compared to other crops.

Pulses, which include beans, lentils, and peas, are considered cancer-friendly for several reasons:

1. **High in Fiber:** Pulses are rich in dietary fiber, which aids in digestion and helps maintain a healthy weight. High-fiber diets have been associated with a reduced risk of certain types of cancer, including colorectal cancer.

2. **Rich in Plant-Based Protein:** Pulses are an excellent source of plant-based protein, which is important for maintaining muscle mass and overall health. Consuming more plant-based protein and less red meat has been linked to a lower risk of cancer.

3. **Antioxidant Properties:** Pulses contain various antioxidants, such as flavonoids and phenolic compounds, which help protect cells from damage caused by free radicals. Antioxidants play a role in reducing inflammation and lowering the risk of cancer development.

4. **Low Glycemic Index:** Pulses have a low glycemic index, meaning they cause a slower and steadier rise in blood sugar levels compared to refined carbohydrates. Diets low in high-glycemic foods may help reduce the risk of certain cancers, including breast and colorectal cancer.

5. **Nutrient-Rich:** Pulses are packed with essential nutrients, including vitamins (such as folate and vitamin B6), minerals (such as iron and magnesium), and phytochemicals, which have protective effects against cancer.

6. **Promote Healthy Weight:** Incorporating pulses into meals can help promote satiety and prevent overeating, which may contribute to maintaining a healthy weight. Obesity is a risk factor for several types of cancer.

7. **Versatile and Easy to Prepare:** Pulses are versatile ingredients that can be used in a variety of dishes, from soups and salads to main courses and snacks. They are also budget-friendly and easy to store, making them accessible for many people.

Overall, including a variety of pulses in your diet as part of a balanced and cancer-friendly eating pattern may contribute to reducing the risk of cancer and promoting overall health.

1. *Lentil and Vegetable Soup:*

- ## *Ingredients:*
    - 1 cup lentils
    - 4 cups vegetable broth
    - 1 onion, chopped
    - 2 carrots, diced
    - 2 celery stalks, chopped
    - 2 cloves garlic, minced
    - 1 teaspoon cumin
    - 1 teaspoon turmeric
    - Salt and pepper to taste

- ## *Instructions:*

1. In a large pot, sauté onions, carrots, and celery until softened.

2. Add garlic, cumin, and turmeric, and cook for another minute.

3. Add lentils and vegetable broth. Bring to a boil, then simmer for 20-25 minutes until lentils are tender.

4. Season with salt and pepper to taste. Serve hot.

2. Chickpea and Spinach Curry:

- **Ingredients:**

  - 1 can chickpeas, drained and rinsed

  - 1 onion, diced

  - 2 cloves garlic, minced

  - 1 teaspoon ginger, grated

  - 1 tablespoon curry powder

  - 1 can diced tomatoes

  - 1 cup coconut milk

  - 2 cups baby spinach

  - Salt and pepper to taste

- **Instructions:**

  1. In a large skillet, sauté onions until translucent. Add garlic and ginger, cook for another minute.

  2. Stir in curry powder and cook until fragrant.

  3. Add diced tomatoes and coconut milk, bring to a simmer.

  4. Add chickpeas and simmer for 10 minutes.

  5. Stir in baby spinach until wilted. Season with salt and pepper. Serve over rice.

3. Black Bean Quesadillas:

- **Ingredients:**

  - 1 can black beans, drained and rinsed

  - 1 bell pepper, diced

- 1 onion, diced

- 1 teaspoon cumin

- 1 teaspoon chili powder

- 4 large tortillas

- 1 cup shredded cheese

- Salsa and guacamole for serving

- ### Instructions:

1. In a skillet, sauté bell pepper and onion until softened.

2. Add black beans, cumin, and chili powder. Cook until heated through.

3. Place a tortilla on a flat surface. Spoon bean mixture onto half of the tortilla, then sprinkle with cheese. Fold the tortilla in half.

4. Cook quesadillas in a skillet over medium heat until golden and crispy on both sides.

5. Slice and serve with salsa and guacamole.

4. Mediterranean Chickpea Salad:

- ### Ingredients:

- 1 can chickpeas, drained and rinsed

- 1 cucumber, diced

- 1 bell pepper, diced

- 1 cup cherry tomatoes, halved

- 1/4 cup red onion, thinly sliced

- 1/4 cup Kalamata olives, sliced

- 2 tablespoons feta cheese, crumbled

- 2 tablespoons olive oil

- 1 tablespoon lemon juice

- 1 teaspoon dried oregano

- Salt and pepper to taste

- *Instructions:*

1. In a large bowl, combine chickpeas, cucumber, bell pepper, tomatoes, red onion, and olives.

2. In a small bowl, whisk together olive oil, lemon juice, oregano, salt, and pepper.

3. Pour dressing over the salad and toss to coat.

4. Sprinkle with feta cheese before serving.

5. Red Lentil Dal:

- *Ingredients:*

- 1 cup red lentils

- 3 cups vegetable broth

- 1 onion, diced

- 2 cloves garlic, minced

- 1 tablespoon ginger, grated

- 1 teaspoon cumin

- 1 teaspoon turmeric

- 1/2 teaspoon garam masala

- 1 can diced tomatoes

- Salt and pepper to taste

- *Instructions:*

    1. In a large pot, sauté onions until translucent. Add garlic and ginger, cook for another minute.

    2. Stir in cumin, turmeric, and garam masala, cook until fragrant.

    3. Add red lentils, vegetable broth, and diced tomatoes. Bring to a boil, then simmer for 20-25 minutes until lentils are soft.

    4. Season with salt and pepper. Serve over rice or with naan bread.

6. White Bean and Kale Soup:

- *Ingredients:*

    - 1 can white beans, drained and rinsed

    - 4 cups vegetable broth

    - 1 onion, chopped

    - 2 carrots, diced

    - 2 celery stalks, chopped

    - 2 cloves garlic, minced

    - 1 teaspoon dried thyme

    - 2 cups chopped kale

    - Salt and pepper to taste

- *Instructions:*

    1. In a large pot, sauté onions, carrots, and celery until softened.

    2. Add garlic and thyme, cook for another minute.

    3. Add white beans and vegetable broth. Bring to a boil, then reduce heat and simmer for 15 minutes.

4. Stir in chopped kale and cook until wilted. Season with salt and pepper. Serve hot.

7. Edamame and Quinoa Salad:

- ***Ingredients:***

  - 1 cup quinoa, cooked

  - 1 cup shelled edamame, cooked

  - 1 bell pepper, diced

  - 1 carrot, grated

  - 1/4 cup fresh cilantro, chopped

  - 2 tablespoons sesame oil

  - 1 tablespoon rice vinegar

  - 1 tablespoon soy sauce

  - 1 teaspoon honey or maple syrup

  - Sesame seeds for garnish

- ***Instructions:***

  1. In a large bowl, combine cooked quinoa, edamame, bell pepper, carrot, and cilantro.

  2. In a small bowl, whisk together sesame oil, rice vinegar, soy sauce, and honey.

  3. Pour dressing over the salad and toss to coat.

  4. Garnish with sesame seeds before serving.

8. Black-Eyed Pea Salad:

- ***Ingredients:***

  - 1 can black-eyed peas, drained and rinsed

- 1 bell pepper, diced

- 1/4 cup red onion, diced

- 1/4 cup fresh parsley, chopped

- 2 tablespoons olive oil

- 1 tablespoon red wine vinegar

- 1 teaspoon Dijon mustard

- Salt and pepper to taste

- *Instructions:*

  1. In a large bowl, combine black-eyed peas, bell pepper, red onion, and parsley.

  2. In a small bowl, whisk together olive oil, red wine vinegar, Dijon mustard, salt, and pepper.

  3. Pour dressing over the salad and toss to coat.

  4. Serve chilled or at room temperature.

9. Spicy Black Bean Tacos:

- *Ingredients:*

  - 1 can black beans, drained and rinsed

  - 1/2 onion, diced

  - 1 clove garlic, minced

  - 1 teaspoon chili powder

  - 1/2 teaspoon cumin

  - Salt and pepper to taste

  - 8 small corn tortillas

- Toppings: avocado, salsa, shredded lettuce, lime wedges

- *Instructions:*

  1. In a skillet, sauté onions and garlic until softened.

  2. Add black beans, chili powder, cumin, salt, and pepper. Cook until heated through.

  3. Heat corn tortillas in a separate skillet until warm and pliable.

  4. Spoon black bean mixture onto each tortilla. Top with avocado, salsa, shredded lettuce, and a squeeze of lime juice.

10. Mushroom and Lentil Shepherd's Pie:

- *Ingredients:*

  - 1 cup green lentils, cooked

  - 2 cups mushrooms, sliced

  - 1 onion, diced

  - 2 carrots, diced

  - 2 cloves garlic, minced

  - 1 teaspoon thyme

  - 1 tablespoon tomato paste

  - 1 cup vegetable broth

  - 2 cups mashed potatoes

  - Salt and pepper to taste

- *Instructions:*

  1. Preheat oven to 375°F (190°C).

2. In a skillet, sauté onions, carrots, and mushrooms until softened.

3. Add garlic, thyme, and tomato paste, cook for another minute.

4. Stir in cooked lentils and vegetable broth. Simmer until thickened.

5. Transfer lentil mixture to a baking dish. Top with mashed potatoes.

6. Bake for 25-30 minutes, or until potatoes are golden brown. Serve hot.

11. Cauliflower and Chickpea Curry:

- ### Ingredients:

    - 1 head cauliflower, cut into florets

    - 1 can chickpeas, drained and rinsed

    - 1 onion, diced

    - 2 cloves garlic, minced

    - 1 tablespoon curry powder

    - 1 teaspoon turmeric

    - 1 can coconut milk

    - 1 can diced tomatoes

    - Salt and pepper to taste

- ### Instructions:

    1. In a large skillet, sauté onions until translucent. Add garlic and cook until fragrant.

    2. Stir in curry powder and turmeric, cook for another minute.

    3. Add cauliflower florets, chickpeas, coconut milk, and diced tomatoes. Bring to a simmer.

    4. Cover and cook for 15-20 minutes, or until cauliflower is tender.

5. Season with salt and pepper. Serve over rice.

12. White Bean and Tomato Bruschetta:

- *Ingredients:*

  - 1 can cannellini beans, drained and rinsed

  - 2 cups cherry tomatoes, halved

  - 1/4 cup red onion, finely chopped

  - 2 cloves garlic, minced

  - 2 tablespoons balsamic vinegar

  - 2 tablespoons olive oil

  - 1 tablespoon fresh basil, chopped

  - Salt and pepper to taste

  - Baguette slices, toasted

- *Instructions:*

  1. In a bowl, combine cannellini beans, cherry tomatoes, red onion, and garlic.

  2. In a small bowl, whisk together balsamic vinegar, olive oil, basil, salt, and pepper.

  3. Pour dressing over the bean mixture and toss to coat.

  4. Spoon bean mixture onto toasted baguette slices. Serve as an appetizer or light meal.

13. Tofu and Vegetable Stir-Fry:

- *Ingredients:*

  - 1 block firm tofu, pressed and cubed

  - 2 cups mixed vegetables (bell peppers, broccoli, snap peas)

- 2 cloves garlic, minced

- 2 tablespoons soy sauce

- 1 tablespoon hoisin sauce

- 1 tablespoon sesame oil

- Cooked brown rice for serving

- ### *Instructions:*

    1. In a large skillet or wok, heat sesame oil over medium heat. Add tofu cubes and cook until golden brown on all sides. Remove from skillet and set aside.

    2. In the same skillet, add mixed vegetables and garlic. Stir-fry until vegetables are tender-crisp.

    3. Return tofu to the skillet. Add soy sauce and hoisin sauce. Cook for another 2-3 minutes, stirring to coat everything evenly.

    4. Serve hot over cooked brown rice.

14. Three-Bean Chili:

- ### *Ingredients:*

    - 1 can black beans, drained and rinsed

    - 1 can kidney beans, drained and rinsed

    - 1 can pinto beans, drained and rinsed

    - 1 onion, diced

    - 2 cloves garlic, minced

    - 1 bell pepper, diced

    - 1 can diced tomatoes

    - 2 tablespoons tomato paste

- 2 teaspoons chili powder

- 1 teaspoon cumin

- Salt and pepper to taste

- **Instructions:**

  1. In a large pot, sauté onions and garlic until softened.

  2. Add bell pepper and cook until slightly tender.

  3. Stir in chili powder and cumin, cook for another minute.

  4. Add diced tomatoes, tomato paste, and drained beans. Bring to a simmer.

  5. Simmer for 20-25 minutes, stirring occasionally.

  6. Season with salt and pepper. Serve hot.

15. Split Pea and Ham Soup:

- **Ingredients:**

  - 1 cup split peas

  - 4 cups chicken or vegetable broth

  - 1 onion, chopped

  - 2 carrots, diced

  - 2 celery stalks, chopped

  - 2 cloves garlic, minced

  - 1 ham hock or ham bone

  - 1 bay leaf

  - Salt and pepper to taste

- **Instructions:**

1. In a large pot, combine split peas, broth, onion, carrots, celery, garlic, ham hock, and bay leaf.

2. Bring to a boil, then reduce heat and simmer for 1.5-2 hours, stirring occasionally, until peas are tender and soup is thickened.

3. Remove ham hock or bone from the soup and discard. Season with salt and pepper.

4. Serve hot, garnished with fresh parsley if desired.

These recipes offer a variety of ways to incorporate beans and legumes into a cancer-friendly diet, providing plenty of nutrients and flavor. Enjoy experimenting with these delicious and nutritious dishes!

CHAPTER 7: SALAD AND DRESSINGS

1. Mixed Greens Salad with Lemon Vinaigrette:

- **Salad Ingredients:**

    - 4 cups mixed greens

    - 1/4 cup cherry tomatoes, halved

    - 1/4 cup cucumber, sliced

    - 2 tablespoons sliced almonds

- **Dressing Ingredients:**

    - 2 tablespoons extra virgin olive oil

    - 1 tablespoon fresh lemon juice

    - 1 teaspoon Dijon mustard

    - 1/2 teaspoon honey

    - Salt and pepper to taste

- **Instructions:**

1. In a large bowl, toss mixed greens, cherry tomatoes, cucumber, and sliced almonds.

2. In a small bowl, whisk together olive oil, lemon juice, Dijon mustard, honey, salt, and pepper until well combined.

3. Drizzle the dressing over the salad just before serving and toss to coat evenly.

2. Kale Caesar Salad with Greek Yogurt Dressing:

- **Salad Ingredients:**

    - 4 cups chopped kale

- 1/4 cup grated Parmesan cheese

- 1/4 cup whole grain croutons

- *Dressing Ingredients:*

  - 1/4 cup Greek yogurt

  - 2 tablespoons lemon juice

  - 1 tablespoon Dijon mustard

  - 1 garlic clove, minced

  - 2 tablespoons grated Parmesan cheese

  - Salt and pepper to taste

- *Instructions:*

  1. In a large bowl, massage the chopped kale with a little olive oil until slightly softened.

  2. Add grated Parmesan cheese and whole grain croutons to the kale.

  3. In a small bowl, whisk together Greek yogurt, lemon juice, Dijon mustard, minced garlic, grated Parmesan cheese, salt, and pepper until smooth.

  4. Drizzle the dressing over the salad and toss to coat well.

3. Spinach Strawberry Salad with Balsamic Glaze:

- *Salad Ingredients:*

  - 4 cups baby spinach leaves

  - 1 cup sliced strawberries

  - 1/4 cup sliced almonds

  - 2 tablespoons crumbled feta cheese

- *Dressing Ingredients:*

  - 2 tablespoons balsamic glaze

  - 1 tablespoon extra virgin olive oil

  - 1 teaspoon honey

  - Salt and pepper to taste

- *Instructions:*

  1. In a large bowl, combine baby spinach leaves, sliced strawberries, sliced almonds, and crumbled feta cheese.

  2. In a small bowl, whisk together balsamic glaze, olive oil, honey, salt, and pepper until well blended.

  3. Drizzle the dressing over the salad just before serving and toss gently to combine.

4. Mango Avocado Quinoa Salad with Lime Dressing:

- *Salad Ingredients:*

  - 2 cups cooked quinoa, cooled

  - 1 ripe mango, diced

  - 1 avocado, diced

  - 1/4 cup chopped cilantro

  - 2 tablespoons pumpkin seeds

- *Dressing Ingredients:*

  - 2 tablespoons fresh lime juice

  - 1 tablespoon honey

  - 1 tablespoon olive oil

- 1/2 teaspoon ground cumin

- Salt and pepper to taste

- ***Instructions:***

  1. In a large bowl, combine cooked quinoa, diced mango, diced avocado, chopped cilantro, and pumpkin seeds.

  2. In a small bowl, whisk together lime juice, honey, olive oil, ground cumin, salt, and pepper until well combined.

  3. Drizzle the dressing over the salad and toss gently to mix all ingredients evenly.

5. Greek Chickpea Salad with Yogurt Tahini Dressing:

- ***Salad Ingredients:***

  - 1 can (15 oz) chickpeas, drained and rinsed

  - 1 cucumber, diced

  - 1 cup cherry tomatoes, halved

  - 1/4 cup diced red onion

  - 1/4 cup chopped fresh parsley

- ***Dressing Ingredients:***

  - 1/4 cup plain Greek yogurt

  - 2 tablespoons tahini

  - 2 tablespoons lemon juice

  - 1 garlic clove, minced

  - 1 tablespoon extra virgin olive oil

  - Salt and pepper to taste

- *Instructions:*

    1. In a large bowl, combine chickpeas, diced cucumber, cherry tomatoes, diced red onion, and chopped fresh parsley.

    2. In a small bowl, whisk together Greek yogurt, tahini, lemon juice, minced garlic, olive oil, salt, and pepper until smooth.

    3. Drizzle the dressing over the salad just before serving and toss gently to coat.

6. Asian Cabbage Salad with Peanut Dressing:

- *Salad Ingredients:*

    - 4 cups shredded cabbage (green or purple)

    - 1 cup shredded carrots

    - 1/4 cup sliced green onions

    - 1/4 cup chopped cilantro

    - 1/4 cup chopped peanuts (optional for garnish)

- *Dressing Ingredients:*

    - 2 tablespoons peanut butter

    - 2 tablespoons soy sauce

    - 1 tablespoon rice vinegar

    - 1 tablespoon honey

    - 1 teaspoon sesame oil

    - 1 garlic clove, minced

    - 1 teaspoon grated ginger

    - 2 tablespoons water (or more as needed)

- *Instructions:*

    1. In a large bowl, combine shredded cabbage, shredded carrots, sliced green onions, and chopped cilantro.

    2. In a small bowl, whisk together peanut butter, soy sauce, rice vinegar, honey, sesame oil, minced garlic, grated ginger, and water until well blended.

    3. If the dressing is too thick, add more water to reach the desired consistency.

    4. Drizzle the peanut dressing over the salad and toss to coat evenly. Sprinkle chopped peanuts on top if desired.

7. Caprese Salad with Balsamic Glaze:

- ### Salad Ingredients:

    - 2 large tomatoes, sliced

    - 1 ball fresh mozzarella cheese, sliced

    - Fresh basil leaves

    - Salt and pepper to taste

- ### Dressing Ingredients:

    - 2 tablespoons balsamic glaze

    - 1 tablespoon extra virgin olive oil

    - 1 teaspoon honey (optional)

- ### Instructions:

    1. Arrange tomato slices and mozzarella cheese slices on a serving plate, alternating them and overlapping slightly.

    2. Tuck fresh basil leaves between the tomato and mozzarella slices.

3. In a small bowl, whisk together balsamic glaze, olive oil, and honey until well combined.

4. Drizzle the dressing over the salad just before serving. Season with salt and pepper to taste.

8. Roasted Vegetable Quinoa Salad with Lemon Herb Dressing:

- **Salad Ingredients:**

  - 2 cups cooked quinoa, cooled

  - 1 cup cherry tomatoes, halved

  - 1 cup diced cucumber

  - 1 cup diced bell peppers (any color)

  - 1/4 cup chopped red onion

  - 1/4 cup crumbled feta cheese

- **Dressing Ingredients:**

  - 3 tablespoons extra virgin olive oil

  - 2 tablespoons fresh lemon juice

  - 1 teaspoon Dijon mustard

  - 1 garlic clove, minced

  - 1 tablespoon chopped fresh herbs (such as basil, parsley, or oregano)

  - Salt and pepper to taste

- **Instructions:**

  1. In a large bowl, combine cooked quinoa, cherry tomatoes, diced cucumber, diced bell peppers, chopped red onion, and crumbled feta cheese.

2. In a small bowl, whisk together olive oil, lemon juice, Dijon mustard, minced garlic, chopped fresh herbs, salt, and pepper until well blended.

3. Drizzle the dressing over the salad and toss gently to mix all ingredients evenly.

9. Grilled Chicken Caesar Salad:

- ### Salad Ingredients:

  - 2 boneless, skinless chicken breasts

  - 4 cups chopped romaine lettuce

  - 1/4 cup grated Parmesan cheese

  - 1/4 cup whole grain croutons

- ### Dressing Ingredients:

  - 1/4 cup plain Greek yogurt

  - 2 tablespoons grated Parmesan cheese

  - 1 tablespoon lemon juice

  - 1 teaspoon Worcestershire sauce

  - 1 garlic clove, minced

  - Salt and pepper to taste

- ### Instructions:

  1. Season the chicken breasts with salt and pepper, then grill or cook in a skillet until cooked through. Let them rest for a few minutes before slicing.

  2. In a large bowl, toss chopped romaine lettuce with grated Parmesan cheese and whole grain croutons.

  3. In a small bowl, whisk together Greek yogurt, grated Parmesan cheese, lemon juice, Worcestershire sauce, minced garlic, salt, and pepper until smooth.

4. Drizzle the dressing over the salad and toss to coat well. Top with sliced grilled chicken breasts before serving.

10. Warm Quinoa and Roasted Vegetable Salad:

- *Salad Ingredients:*

  - 2 cups cooked quinoa, warm

  - 1 cup roasted vegetables (such as carrots, bell peppers, zucchini, and red onion)

  - 1/4 cup chopped fresh parsley

  - 2 tablespoons toasted pine nuts

- *Dressing Ingredients:*

  - 3 tablespoons extra virgin olive oil

  - 2 tablespoons balsamic vinegar

  - 1 teaspoon Dijon mustard

  - 1 garlic clove, minced

  - Salt and pepper to taste

- *Instructions:*

  1. In a large bowl, combine warm cooked quinoa, roasted vegetables, chopped fresh parsley, and toasted pine nuts.

  2. In a small bowl, whisk together olive oil, balsamic vinegar, Dijon mustard, minced garlic, salt, and pepper until well blended.

  3. Drizzle the dressing over the salad and toss gently to mix all ingredients evenly.

11. Tuna White Bean Salad with Lemon Herb Dressing:

- **Salad Ingredients:**

- 1 can (5 oz) tuna, drained

- 1 can (15 oz) cannellini beans, drained and rinsed

- 1/4 cup diced red onion

- 1/4 cup chopped fresh parsley

- 1/4 cup chopped cherry tomatoes

- **Dressing Ingredients:**

  - 2 tablespoons fresh lemon juice

  - 2 tablespoons extra virgin olive oil

  - 1 garlic clove, minced

  - 1 teaspoon Dijon mustard

  - 1 tablespoon chopped fresh herbs (such as dill, parsley, or chives)

  - Salt and pepper to taste

- **Instructions:**

  1. In a large bowl, combine drained tuna, cannellini beans, diced red onion, chopped fresh parsley, and chopped cherry tomatoes.

  2. In a small bowl, whisk together fresh lemon juice, olive oil, minced garlic, Dijon mustard, chopped fresh herbs, salt, and pepper until well combined.

  3. Drizzle the dressing over the salad and toss gently to coat all ingredients evenly.

12. Beet and Goat Cheese Salad with Orange Balsamic Dressing:

- **Salad Ingredients:**

  - 2 medium beets, cooked and sliced

- 4 cups mixed salad greens

- 1/4 cup crumbled goat cheese

- 1/4 cup toasted walnuts

- *Dressing Ingredients:*

  - 2 tablespoons orange juice

  - 2 tablespoons balsamic vinegar

  - 1 tablespoon honey

  - 2 tablespoons extra virgin olive oil

  - Salt and pepper to taste

- *Instructions:*

  1. Arrange cooked and sliced beets over mixed salad greens in a serving bowl.

  2. Sprinkle crumbled goat cheese and toasted walnuts over the beets and greens.

  3. In a small bowl, whisk together orange juice, balsamic vinegar, honey, olive oil, salt, and pepper until well blended.

  4. Drizzle the dressing over the salad just before serving and toss gently to coat.

13. Broccoli and Quinoa Salad with Lemon Tahini Dressing:

- *Salad Ingredients:*

  - 2 cups cooked quinoa, cooled

  - 2 cups steamed broccoli florets, cooled

  - 1/4 cup dried cranberries

  - 1/4 cup chopped almonds

- **Dressing Ingredients:**

- 1/4 cup tahini

- 2 tablespoons fresh lemon juice

- 1 tablespoon honey

- 1 garlic clove, minced

- 2-4 tablespoons water (as needed)

- Salt and pepper to taste

- **Instructions:**

  1. In a large bowl, combine cooked quinoa, steamed broccoli florets, dried cranberries, and chopped almonds.

  2. In a small bowl, whisk together tahini, fresh lemon juice, honey, minced garlic, salt, and pepper. Thin the dressing with water to achieve desired consistency.

  3. Drizzle the lemon tahini dressing over the salad and toss gently to coat all ingredients evenly.

14. Pear and Walnut Salad with Honey Mustard Dressing:

- **Salad Ingredients:**

  - 4 cups mixed salad greens

  - 1 ripe pear, sliced

  - 1/4 cup crumbled blue cheese

  - 1/4 cup chopped walnuts, toasted

- **Dressing Ingredients:**

  - 2 tablespoons extra virgin olive oil

  - 1 tablespoon apple cider vinegar

  - 1 teaspoon Dijon mustard

- 1 teaspoon honey

- Salt and pepper to taste

- **Instructions:**

  1. Arrange mixed salad greens on a serving plate. Top with sliced pear, crumbled blue cheese, and toasted chopped walnuts.

  2. In a small bowl, whisk together olive oil, apple cider vinegar, Dijon mustard, honey, salt, and pepper until well combined.

  3. Drizzle the honey mustard dressing over the salad just before serving and toss gently to coat.

15. Roasted Cauliflower Salad with Tahini Turmeric Dressing:

- ### *Salad Ingredients:*

  - 1 small head cauliflower, cut into florets

  - 2 tablespoons olive oil

  - Salt and pepper to taste

  - 4 cups baby spinach leaves

  - 1/4 cup dried cranberries

  - 1/4 cup toasted pumpkin seeds

- ### *Dressing Ingredients:*

  - 1/4 cup tahini

  - 2 tablespoons fresh lemon juice

  - 1 teaspoon ground turmeric

  - 1 garlic clove, minced

  - 2-4 tablespoons water (as needed)

- Salt and pepper to taste

- ***Instructions***:

  1. Preheat the oven to 400°F (200°C). Toss cauliflower florets with olive oil, salt, and pepper. Spread them on a baking sheet and roast for 20-25 minutes, until golden brown and tender.

  2. In a large bowl, combine roasted cauliflower florets with baby spinach leaves, dried cranberries, and toasted pumpkin seeds.

  3. In a small bowl, whisk together tahini, fresh lemon juice, ground turmeric, minced garlic, salt, and pepper. Thin the dressing with water to achieve desired consistency.

  4. Drizzle the tahini turmeric dressing over the salad and toss gently to coat all ingredients evenly.

These salad recipes offer a variety of flavors and textures while incorporating cancer-fighting ingredients and nutritious dressings. Enjoy experimenting with different combinations to find your favorites!

CHAPTER 8: SOUPS AND STEW

1. Chicken and Vegetable Soup:

- ### Ingredients:

  - 1 tablespoon olive oil

  - 1 onion, diced

  - 2 carrots, sliced

  - 2 celery stalks, sliced

  - 2 cloves garlic, minced

  - 6 cups low-sodium chicken broth

  - 2 cups cooked chicken breast, shredded

  - 1 cup chopped spinach

  - Salt and pepper to taste

- ### Instructions:

1. Heat olive oil in a large pot over medium heat. Add onion, carrots, and celery. Cook until softened, about 5 minutes.

2. Add minced garlic and cook for another minute.

3. Pour in chicken broth and bring to a simmer.

4. Add shredded chicken and chopped spinach. Simmer for 10-15 minutes.

5. Season with salt and pepper to taste before serving.

2. Vegetable Lentil Soup:

- *Ingredients:*

  - 1 tablespoon olive oil

  - 1 onion, diced

  - 2 carrots, diced

  - 2 celery stalks, diced

  - 2 cloves garlic, minced

  - 1 cup dried lentils, rinsed

  - 6 cups vegetable broth

  - 1 can (14 oz) diced tomatoes

  - 1 teaspoon dried thyme

  - Salt and pepper to taste

- *Instructions:*

  1. Heat olive oil in a large pot over medium heat. Add onion, carrots, and celery. Cook until softened, about 5 minutes.

  2. Add minced garlic and cook for another minute.

  3. Add dried lentils, vegetable broth, diced tomatoes, and dried thyme. Bring to a boil, then reduce heat and simmer for 20-25 minutes, or until lentils are tender.

  4. Season with salt and pepper to taste before serving.

3. Butternut Squash Soup:

- *Ingredients:*

  - 1 butternut squash, peeled, seeded, and diced

  - 1 onion, diced

- 2 carrots, diced

- 2 celery stalks, diced

- 4 cups vegetable broth

- 1 teaspoon ground cumin

- 1/2 teaspoon ground cinnamon

- Salt and pepper to taste

- **Instructions:**

  1. In a large pot, combine butternut squash, onion, carrots, celery, and vegetable broth.

  2. Bring to a boil, then reduce heat and simmer until vegetables are tender, about 20 minutes.

  3. Use an immersion blender to puree the soup until smooth. Alternatively, transfer the soup to a blender and puree in batches.

  4. Stir in ground cumin and ground cinnamon. Season with salt and pepper to taste before serving.

4. Tomato Basil Soup:

- **Ingredients:**

  - 1 tablespoon olive oil

  - 1 onion, diced

  - 2 cloves garlic, minced

  - 1 can (28 oz) diced tomatoes

  - 2 cups vegetable broth

  - 1/4 cup chopped fresh basil

- Salt and pepper to taste

- *Instructions:*

  1. Heat olive oil in a large pot over medium heat. Add onion and cook until softened, about 5 minutes.

  2. Add minced garlic and cook for another minute.

  3. Pour in diced tomatoes and vegetable broth. Bring to a simmer and cook for 15-20 minutes.

  4. Use an immersion blender to puree the soup until smooth. Alternatively, transfer the soup to a blender and puree in batches.

  5. Stir in chopped fresh basil. Season with salt and pepper to taste before serving.

5. Mushroom Barley Soup:

- *Ingredients:*

  - 1 tablespoon olive oil

  - 1 onion, diced

  - 2 carrots, diced

  - 2 celery stalks, diced

  - 8 oz mushrooms, sliced

  - 1/2 cup pearl barley

  - 6 cups vegetable broth

  - 1 teaspoon dried thyme

  - Salt and pepper to taste

- *Instructions:*

1. Heat olive oil in a large pot over medium heat. Add onion, carrots, celery, and mushrooms. Cook until softened, about 5-7 minutes.

2. Add pearl barley and vegetable broth. Bring to a boil, then reduce heat and simmer for 40-45 minutes, or until barley is tender.

3. Stir in dried thyme. Season with salt and pepper to taste before serving.

6. Spinach and White Bean Soup:

- ### Ingredients:

  - 1 tablespoon olive oil

  - 1 onion, diced

  - 2 carrots, diced

  - 2 celery stalks, diced

  - 2 cloves garlic, minced

  - 6 cups vegetable broth

  - 2 cans (15 oz each) white beans, drained and rinsed

  - 4 cups chopped spinach

  - 1 teaspoon dried oregano

  - Salt and pepper to taste

- ### Instructions:

  1. Heat olive oil in a large pot over medium heat. Add onion, carrots, celery, and garlic. Cook until softened, about 5 minutes.

  2. Add vegetable broth, white beans, chopped spinach, and dried oregano. Bring to a simmer and cook for 15-20 minutes.

3. Use an immersion blender to partially puree the soup, leaving some beans and vegetables whole. Alternatively, transfer a portion of the soup to a blender and puree, then return it to the pot.

4. Season with salt and pepper to taste before serving.

7. Turmeric Lentil Soup:

- ## *Ingredients:*

  - 1 tablespoon olive oil

  - 1 onion, diced

  - 2 carrots, diced

  - 2 celery stalks, diced

  - 2 cloves garlic, minced

  - 1 teaspoon ground turmeric

  - 1 cup dried red lentils, rinsed

  - 6 cups vegetable broth

  - 1 lemon, juiced

  - Salt and pepper to taste

- ## *Instructions:*

  1. Heat olive oil in a large pot over medium heat. Add onion, carrots, celery, and garlic. Cook until softened, about 5 minutes.

  2. Stir in ground turmeric and cook for another minute.

  3. Add dried red lentils and vegetable broth. Bring to a boil, then reduce heat and simmer for 20-25 minutes, or until lentils are tender.

  4. Stir in lemon juice. Season with salt and pepper to taste before serving.

8. Broccoli Cheddar Soup:

- ### Ingredients:

  - 2 tablespoons butter

  - 1 onion, diced

  - 2 carrots, diced

  - 2 celery stalks, diced

  - 2 cloves garlic, minced

  - 4 cups chopped broccoli florets

  - 4 cups vegetable broth

  - 1 cup shredded cheddar cheese

  - 1 cup milk

  - Salt and pepper to taste

- ### Instructions:

  1. In a large pot, melt butter over medium heat. Add onion, carrots, celery, and garlic. Cook until softened, about 5 minutes.

  2. Add chopped broccoli florets and vegetable broth. Bring to a simmer and cook for 15-20 minutes, or until broccoli is tender.

  3. Use an immersion blender to puree the soup until smooth. Alternatively, transfer the soup to a blender and puree in batches.

  4. Stir in shredded cheddar cheese and milk until cheese is melted and soup is heated through.

  5. Season with salt and pepper to taste before serving.

9. Thai Coconut Curry Soup:

- *Ingredients:*

  - 1 tablespoon olive oil

  - 1 onion, diced

  - 2 carrots, diced

  - 2 cloves garlic, minced

  - 2 tablespoons Thai red curry paste

  - 4 cups vegetable broth

  - 1 can (14 oz) coconut milk

  - 2 cups chopped mixed vegetables (such as bell peppers, zucchini, and mushrooms)

  - 1 tablespoon soy sauce

  - 1 tablespoon brown sugar

  - Salt and pepper to taste

  - Fresh cilantro for garnish

- *Instructions:*

  1. Heat olive oil in a large pot over medium heat. Add onion, carrots, and garlic. Cook until softened, about 5 minutes.

  2. Stir in Thai red curry paste and cook for another minute.

  3. Add vegetable broth, coconut milk, mixed vegetables, soy sauce, and brown sugar. Bring to a simmer and cook for 15-20 minutes.

  4. Season with salt and pepper to taste. Garnish with fresh cilantro before serving.

10. Moroccan Chickpea Stew:

- *Ingredients:*

- 1 tablespoon olive oil

- 1 onion, diced

- 2 carrots, diced

- 2 celery stalks, diced

- 2 cloves garlic, minced

- 1 teaspoon ground cumin

- 1 teaspoon ground coriander

- 1/2 teaspoon ground cinnamon

- 1/4 teaspoon ground ginger

- 1 can (15 oz) chickpeas, drained and rinsed

- 1 can (14 oz) diced tomatoes

- 4 cups vegetable broth

- 1/4 cup chopped fresh cilantro

- Salt and pepper to taste

- ***Instructions:***

1. Heat olive oil in a large pot over medium heat. Add onion, carrots, celery, and garlic. Cook until softened, about 5 minutes.

2. Stir in ground cumin, ground coriander, ground cinnamon, and ground ginger. Cook for another minute.

3. Add chickpeas, diced tomatoes, and vegetable broth. Bring to a simmer and cook for 20-25 minutes.

4. Stir in chopped fresh cilantro. Season with salt and pepper to taste before serving.

11. Italian Minestrone Soup:

- *Ingredients:*

  - 1 tablespoon olive oil

  - 1 onion, diced

  - 2 carrots, diced

  - 2 celery stalks, diced

  - 2 cloves garlic, minced

  - 1 can (15 oz) kidney beans, drained and rinsed

  - 1 can (14 oz) diced tomatoes

  - 4 cups vegetable broth

  - 1 cup small pasta (such as ditalini or small shells)

  - 2 cups chopped spinach

  - 1 teaspoon dried basil

  - 1 teaspoon dried oregano

  - Salt and pepper to taste

- *Instructions:*

  1. Heat olive oil in a large pot over medium heat. Add onion, carrots, celery, and garlic. Cook until softened, about 5 minutes.

  2. Add kidney beans, diced tomatoes, vegetable broth, pasta, dried basil, and dried oregano. Bring to a boil, then reduce heat and simmer for 10-12 minutes, or until pasta is cooked.

  3. Stir in chopped spinach and cook until wilted. Season with salt and pepper to taste before serving.

12. Cauliflower and Leek Soup:

- *Ingredients:*

  - 1 tablespoon olive oil

  - 2 leeks, white and light green parts only, sliced

  - 1 head cauliflower, chopped

  - 4 cups vegetable broth

  - 1 teaspoon dried thyme

  - Salt and pepper to taste

  - Fresh chives for garnish

- *Instructions:*

  1. Heat olive oil in a large pot over medium heat. Add sliced leeks and cook until softened, about 5 minutes.

  2. Add chopped cauliflower, vegetable broth, and dried thyme. Bring to a boil, then reduce heat and simmer for 20-25 minutes, or until cauliflower is tender.

  3. Use an immersion blender to puree the soup until smooth. Alternatively, transfer the soup to a blender and puree in batches.

  4. Season with salt and pepper to taste. Garnish with fresh chives before serving.

13. Split Pea Soup:

- *Ingredients:*

  - 1 tablespoon olive oil

  - 1 onion, diced

  - 2 carrots, diced

  - 2 celery stalks, diced

  - 2 cloves garlic, minced

- 1 bay leaf

- 1 teaspoon dried thyme

- 1 cup dried split peas, rinsed

- 4 cups vegetable broth

- Salt and pepper to taste

- **Instructions:**

  1. Heat olive oil in a large pot over medium heat. Add onion, carrots, celery, and garlic. Cook until softened, about 5 minutes.

  2. Add bay leaf, dried thyme, dried split peas, and vegetable broth. Bring to a boil, then reduce heat and simmer for 40-45 minutes, or until split peas are tender.

  3. Remove the bay leaf. Use an immersion blender to partially puree the soup, leaving some split peas whole. Alternatively, transfer a portion of the soup to a blender and puree, then return it to the pot.

  4. Season with salt and pepper to taste before serving.

14. Spicy Black Bean Soup:

- **Ingredients:**

  - 1 tablespoon olive oil

  - 1 onion, diced

  - 2 cloves garlic, minced

  - 1 red bell pepper, diced

  - 2 teaspoons chili powder

  - 1 teaspoon ground cumin

  - 1/2 teaspoon smoked paprika

- 2 cans (15 oz each) black beans, drained and rinsed

- 4 cups vegetable broth

- 1 can (14 oz) diced tomatoes

- Salt and pepper to taste

- Fresh cilantro for garnish

- ***Instructions:***

  1. Heat olive oil in a large pot over medium heat. Add onion, garlic, and red bell pepper. Cook until softened, about 5 minutes.

  2. Stir in chili powder, ground cumin, and smoked paprika. Cook for another minute.

  3. Add black beans, vegetable broth, and diced tomatoes. Bring to a simmer and cook for 15-20 minutes.

  4. Use an immersion blender to partially puree the soup, leaving some black beans whole. Alternatively, transfer a portion of the soup to a blender and puree, then return it to the pot.

  5. Season with salt and pepper to taste. Garnish with fresh cilantro before serving.

15. Coconut Lentil Curry:

- ***Ingredients:***

  - 1 tablespoon olive oil

  - 1 onion, diced

  - 2 cloves garlic, minced

  - 1 tablespoon grated fresh ginger

  - 1 tablespoon curry powder

  - 1 cup dried red lentils, rinsed

- 1 can (14 oz) diced tomatoes

- 1 can (14 oz) coconut milk

- 2 cups vegetable broth

- 2 cups chopped spinach

- Salt and pepper to taste

- Fresh cilantro for garnish

- *Instructions:*

1. Heat olive oil in a large pot over medium heat. Add onion and cook until softened, about 5 minutes.

2. Add minced garlic, grated fresh ginger, and curry powder. Cook for another minute.

3. Add dried red lentils, diced tomatoes, coconut milk, and vegetable broth. Bring to a boil, then reduce heat and simmer for 20-25 minutes, or until lentils are tender.

4. Stir in chopped spinach and cook until wilted. Season with salt and pepper to taste.

5. Garnish with fresh cilantro before serving.

Enjoy these comforting and nutritious soup and stew recipes!

CHAPTER 9: SMOOTHIES

1. Green Detox Smoothie:

- **Ingredients:**

  - 1 cup spinach

  - 1/2 cup kale

  - 1/2 cucumber, peeled and chopped

  - 1 green apple, cored and chopped

  - 1/2 lemon, juiced

  - 1 tablespoon fresh ginger, grated

  - 1 cup coconut water

  - Optional: 1 tablespoon chia seeds

- **Instructions:**

1. Combine all ingredients in a blender.

2. Blend until smooth.

3. Add more coconut water if needed for desired consistency.

4. Serve immediately and enjoy!

2. Berry Antioxidant Smoothie:

- **Ingredients:**

  - 1/2 cup mixed berries (strawberries, blueberries, raspberries)

  - 1/2 banana

  - 1/2 cup spinach

- 1/4 cup Greek yogurt

- 1 tablespoon flaxseeds

- 1/2 cup almond milk

- *Instructions:*

  1. Place all ingredients in a blender.

  2. Blend until smooth.

  3. Adjust consistency by adding more almond milk if necessary.

  4. Pour into a glass and enjoy!

3. Turmeric Mango Smoothie:

- *Ingredients:*

  - 1 cup frozen mango chunks

  - 1/2 banana

  - 1/2 teaspoon ground turmeric

  - 1/4 teaspoon ground cinnamon

  - 1 tablespoon honey or maple syrup

  - 1/2 cup coconut water

- *Instructions:*

  1. Combine all ingredients in a blender.

  2. Blend until smooth.

  3. Taste and adjust sweetness if necessary.

  4. Pour into a glass and serve immediately.

4. Pineapple Ginger Smoothie:

- *Ingredients:*

  - 1 cup pineapple chunks

  - 1/2 banana

  - 1 tablespoon fresh ginger, grated

  - 1/4 cup Greek yogurt

  - 1/2 cup coconut water

  - Handful of ice cubes

- *Instructions:*

  1. Place all ingredients in a blender.

  2. Blend until smooth.

  3. Add more coconut water if needed to reach desired consistency.

  4. Pour into glasses and garnish with a pineapple wedge if desired.

5. Avocado Banana Smoothie:

- *Ingredients:*

  - 1/2 ripe avocado

  - 1/2 banana

  - 1 cup spinach

  - 1 tablespoon honey or maple syrup

  - 1/2 cup almond milk

- *Instructions:*

  1. Combine all ingredients in a blender.

  2. Blend until smooth and creamy.

3. Add more almond milk if needed to reach desired consistency.

4. Pour into a glass and enjoy!

6. Tropical Coconut Smoothie:

- **Ingredients:**

  - 1/2 cup frozen pineapple chunks

  - 1/2 cup frozen mango chunks

  - 1/2 banana

  - 1/4 cup Greek yogurt

  - 1/4 cup coconut milk

  - Handful of spinach (optional)

- **Instructions:**

  1. Add all ingredients to a blender.

  2. Blend until smooth and creamy.

  3. Adjust thickness by adding more coconut milk if needed.

  4. Pour into glasses and serve with a slice of pineapple for garnish.

7. Blueberry Kale Smoothie:

- **Ingredients:**

  - 1/2 cup blueberries (fresh or frozen)

  - 1/2 cup chopped kale

  - 1/2 banana

  - 1 tablespoon almond butter

- 1 tablespoon chia seeds

- 1/2 cup almond milk

- *Instructions:*

    1. Combine all ingredients in a blender.

    2. Blend until smooth and creamy.

    3. Add more almond milk if necessary to reach desired consistency.

    4. Pour into glasses and serve immediately.

8. Strawberry Banana Spinach Smoothie:

- *Ingredients:*

    - 1/2 cup strawberries (fresh or frozen)

    - 1/2 banana

    - 1 cup spinach

    - 1/4 cup Greek yogurt

    - 1/2 cup almond milk

    - 1 tablespoon honey or maple syrup

- *Instructions:*

    1. Place all ingredients in a blender.

    2. Blend until smooth and creamy.

    3. Adjust sweetness with honey or maple syrup if desired.

    4. Pour into glasses and enjoy!

9. Chocolate Avocado Smoothie:

- *Ingredients:*

  - 1/2 ripe avocado

  - 1 tablespoon unsweetened cocoa powder

  - 1/2 banana

  - 1 tablespoon honey or maple syrup

  - 1/2 cup almond milk

  - Handful of ice cubes

- *Instructions:*

  1. Combine all ingredients in a blender.

  2. Blend until smooth and creamy.

  3. Add more almond milk if needed for desired consistency.

  4. Pour into glasses and serve with a sprinkle of cocoa powder on top.

10. Vanilla Berry Protein Smoothie:

- *Ingredients:*

  - 1/2 cup mixed berries (strawberries, blueberries, raspberries)

  - 1/2 banana

  - 1 scoop vanilla protein powder

  - 1 tablespoon almond butter

  - 1/2 cup almond milk

- *Instructions:*

  1. Place all ingredients in a blender.

  2. Blend until smooth and creamy.

3. Adjust consistency by adding more almond milk if needed.

4. Pour into glasses and enjoy as a post-workout refuel.

11. Mango Coconut Chia Smoothie:

- **Ingredients:**

  - 1/2 cup frozen mango chunks

  - 1/2 banana

  - 1 tablespoon chia seeds

  - 1/4 cup coconut milk

  - 1/2 cup coconut water

  - Handful of spinach (optional)

- **Instructions:**

  1. Combine all ingredients in a blender.

  2. Blend until smooth and creamy.

  3. Add more coconut water if needed to adjust consistency.

  4. Pour into glasses and garnish with shredded coconut if desired.

12. Peach Almond Smoothie:

- **Ingredients:**

  - 1 ripe peach, pitted and chopped

  - 1/2 banana

  - 1/4 cup Greek yogurt

  - 1 tablespoon almond butter

- 1/2 cup almond milk

- Handful of ice cubes

- *Instructions:*

  1. Add all ingredients to a blender.

  2. Blend until smooth and creamy.

  3. Adjust sweetness with honey or maple syrup if desired.

  4. Pour into glasses and enjoy!

13. Citrus Carrot Smoothie:

- *Ingredients:*

  - 1 orange, peeled and segmented

  - 1/2 cup chopped carrots

  - 1/2 banana

  - 1/4 cup Greek yogurt

  - 1/2 cup orange juice

  - Handful of ice cubes

- *Instructions:*

  1. Combine all ingredients in a blender.

  2. Blend until smooth and creamy.

  3. Add more orange juice if needed to adjust consistency.

  4. Pour into glasses and serve with a slice of orange for garnish.

14. Pineapple Mint Smoothie:

- *Ingredients:*

  - 1 cup frozen pineapple chunks

  - 1/2 banana

  - 1/4 cup fresh mint leaves

  - 1/2 cup coconut water

  - Juice of 1/2 lime

  - Handful of ice cubes

- *Instructions:*

  1. Place all ingredients in a blender.

  2. Blend until smooth and creamy.

  3. Adjust sweetness with honey or maple syrup if desired.

  4. Pour into glasses and garnish with a sprig of mint.

15. Raspberry Almond Smoothie:

- *Ingredients:*

  - 1/2 cup raspberries (fresh or frozen)

  - 1/2 banana

  - 1 tablespoon almond butter

  - 1/4 cup Greek yogurt

  - 1/2 cup almond milk

  - Handful of ice cubes

- *Instructions:*

  1. Add all ingredients to a blender.

2. Blend until smooth and creamy.

3. Adjust consistency by adding more almond milk if needed.

4. Pour into glasses and serve with a few whole raspberries on top.

Enjoy these delicious and nutritious smoothie recipes as part of your cancer-friendly diet!

CHAPTER 10: SNACKS AND DESSERTS

1. Chia Seed Pudding:

- ### Ingredients:

  - 1/4 cup chia seeds

  - 1 cup unsweetened almond milk

  - 1 tablespoon honey or maple syrup

  - Fresh fruits for topping (e.g., berries, sliced banana)

- ### Instructions:

1. In a bowl or jar, mix chia seeds, almond milk, and honey or maple syrup.

2. Stir well, cover, and refrigerate for at least 2 hours or overnight until thickened.

3. Serve chilled with fresh fruits on top.

2. Homemade Trail Mix:

- ### Ingredients:

  - 1/2 cup almonds

  - 1/2 cup walnuts

  - 1/4 cup pumpkin seeds

  - 1/4 cup dried cranberries

  - 1/4 cup dark chocolate chips

- ### Instructions:

  1. Mix all ingredients in a bowl.

2. Store in an airtight container for a quick and healthy snack.

3. Greek Yogurt with Honey and Nuts:

- **Ingredients:**

  - 1/2 cup Greek yogurt

  - 1 tablespoon honey

  - 2 tablespoons chopped nuts (e.g., almonds, walnuts)

- **Instructions:**

  1. Place Greek yogurt in a bowl.

  2. Drizzle with honey and sprinkle chopped nuts on top.

  3. Enjoy as a satisfying and protein-rich snack.

4. Baked Apple Chips:

- **Ingredients:**

  - 2 apples, thinly sliced

  - 1 tablespoon lemon juice

  - 1/2 teaspoon cinnamon

- **Instructions:**

  1. Preheat oven to 200°F (93°C) and line a baking sheet with parchment paper.

  2. Toss apple slices with lemon juice and cinnamon in a bowl.

  3. Arrange apple slices on the baking sheet in a single layer.

  4. Bake for 1.5 to 2 hours, flipping halfway through, until apples are dried and crispy.

  5. Allow to cool before serving.

5. Banana Oat Cookies:

- **Ingredients:**
  - 2 ripe bananas, mashed
  - 1 cup rolled oats
  - 1/4 cup chopped nuts (e.g., almonds, pecans)
  - 1/4 cup dried fruit (e.g., raisins, chopped dates)
  - 1/2 teaspoon cinnamon

- **Instructions:**
  1. Preheat oven to 350°F (175°C) and line a baking sheet with parchment paper.
  2. In a bowl, combine mashed bananas, rolled oats, chopped nuts, dried fruit, and cinnamon.
  3. Drop spoonfuls of the mixture onto the baking sheet and flatten slightly with the back of a spoon.
  4. Bake for 15-18 minutes or until golden brown.
  5. Allow to cool before serving.

6. Edamame Hummus with Veggie Sticks:

- **Ingredients:**
  - 1 cup shelled edamame (cooked)
  - 1 clove garlic, minced
  - 2 tablespoons tahini
  - 2 tablespoons lemon juice
  - 2 tablespoons olive oil

- Salt and pepper to taste

- Assorted vegetable sticks (carrots, cucumbers, bell peppers) for dipping

- *Instructions:*

  1. In a food processor, combine edamame, garlic, tahini, lemon juice, and olive oil.

  2. Blend until smooth, adding water if needed to reach desired consistency.

  3. Season with salt and pepper to taste.

  4. Serve with vegetable sticks for dipping.

7. Coconut Date Energy Balls:

- *Ingredients:*

  - 1 cup Medjool dates, pitted

  - 1 cup rolled oats

  - 1/2 cup shredded coconut (unsweetened)

  - 2 tablespoons almond butter

  - 1 tablespoon chia seeds

  - 1/2 teaspoon vanilla extract

- *Instructions:*

  1. Place dates in a food processor and pulse until chopped into small pieces.

  2. Add rolled oats, shredded coconut, almond butter, chia seeds, and vanilla extract to the food processor.

  3. Process until the mixture comes together and forms a sticky dough.

  4. Roll the dough into small balls using your hands.

  5. Optional: Roll the balls in additional shredded coconut for coating.

6. Refrigerate for at least 30 minutes before serving.

8. Stuffed Bell Peppers with Quinoa and Black Beans:

- ## Ingredients:

  - 2 bell peppers, halved and seeds removed

  - 1/2 cup cooked quinoa

  - 1/2 cup black beans, drained and rinsed

  - 1/4 cup corn kernels

  - 1/4 cup diced tomatoes

  - 1/4 cup diced avocado

  - 2 tablespoons chopped cilantro

  - Juice of 1 lime

  - Salt and pepper to taste

- ## Instructions:

  1. Preheat oven to 375°F (190°C) and line a baking dish with parchment paper.

  2. In a bowl, combine cooked quinoa, black beans, corn, tomatoes, avocado, cilantro, lime juice, salt, and pepper.

  3. Stuff each bell pepper half with the quinoa mixture.

  4. Place stuffed peppers in the baking dish and cover with foil.

  5. Bake for 25-30 minutes, or until peppers are tender.

  6. Serve warm as a nutritious snack or light meal.

9. Cucumber and Hummus Bites:

- ## Ingredients:

- 1 cucumber, sliced into rounds

- 1/2 cup hummus

- Cherry tomatoes for garnish

- Fresh parsley for garnish

- ### Instructions:

  1. Spread a small amount of hummus onto each cucumber round.

  2. Top with a cherry tomato and a small sprig of parsley.

  3. Arrange on a serving platter and enjoy as a refreshing snack.

10. Berry Yogurt Bark:

- ### Ingredients:

  - 1 cup Greek yogurt

  - 1 tablespoon honey or maple syrup

  - 1/2 cup mixed berries (strawberries, blueberries, raspberries)

  - 2 tablespoons granola (optional)

- ### Instructions:

  1. Line a baking sheet with parchment paper.

  2. In a bowl, mix Greek yogurt with honey or maple syrup.

  3. Spread the yogurt mixture evenly onto the parchment paper.

  4. Sprinkle mixed berries and granola over the yogurt.

  5. Freeze for 2-3 hours or until firm.

  6. Break into pieces and enjoy as a healthy frozen treat.

11. Avocado Chocolate Mousse:

- *Ingredients:*

  - 2 ripe avocados

  - 1/4 cup cocoa powder

  - 1/4 cup honey or maple syrup

  - 1 teaspoon vanilla extract

  - Pinch of salt

- *Instructions:*

  1. Scoop the flesh of the avocados into a food processor.

  2. Add cocoa powder, honey or maple syrup, vanilla extract, and salt.

  3. Blend until smooth and creamy, scraping down the sides as needed.

  4. Transfer to serving bowls and refrigerate until chilled.

  5. Serve topped with fresh berries or shredded coconut if desired.

12. Spinach and Feta Stuffed Mushrooms:

- *Ingredients:*

  - 8 large mushrooms, stems removed

  - 1 cup chopped spinach

  - 1/4 cup crumbled feta cheese

  - 2 tablespoons chopped sun-dried tomatoes

  - 1 clove garlic, minced

  - Salt and pepper to taste

  - Olive oil for brushing

- *Instructions:*

1. Preheat oven to 375°F (190°C) and line a baking sheet with parchment paper.

2. In a bowl, mix together chopped spinach, feta cheese, sun-dried tomatoes, garlic, salt, and pepper.

3. Spoon the spinach mixture into each mushroom cap.

4. Place stuffed mushrooms on the baking sheet and lightly brush with olive oil.

5. Bake for 15-20 minutes, or until mushrooms are tender.

6. Serve warm as a tasty appetizer or snack.

13. Frozen Banana Pops:

- **Ingredients:**

  - 2 ripe bananas, peeled and cut in half

  - 1/4 cup dark chocolate chips

  - 2 tablespoons unsweetened shredded coconut

  - 2 tablespoons chopped nuts (e.g., almonds, peanuts)

  - Wooden popsicle sticks

- **Instructions:**

  1. Insert a wooden popsicle stick into each banana half.

  2. Place bananas on a parchment-lined baking sheet and freeze until firm.

  3. Melt dark chocolate chips in the microwave or over a double boiler until smooth.

  4. Dip each frozen banana half into the melted chocolate, then sprinkle with shredded coconut and chopped nuts.

  5. Place back on the baking sheet and freeze until the chocolate sets.

  6. Enjoy these refreshing treats straight from the freezer.

14. Roasted Chickpeas:

- **Ingredients:**

    - 1 can (15 ounces) chickpeas (garbanzo beans), drained and rinsed

    - 1 tablespoon olive oil

    - 1 teaspoon ground cumin

    - 1/2 teaspoon smoked paprika

    - 1/2 teaspoon garlic powder

    - Salt to taste

- **Instructions:**

    1. Preheat oven to 400°F (200°C) and line a baking sheet with parchment paper.

    2. Pat the chickpeas dry with a paper towel and remove any loose skins.

    3. In a bowl, toss chickpeas with olive oil, ground cumin, smoked paprika, garlic powder, and salt until evenly coated.

    4. Spread chickpeas in a single layer on the prepared baking sheet.

    5. Roast for 25-30 minutes, shaking the pan halfway through, until chickpeas are crispy and golden brown.

    6. Allow to cool slightly before serving as a crunchy and protein-packed snack.

15. Spinach and Artichoke Dip:

- **Ingredients:**

    - 1 can (14 ounces) artichoke hearts, drained and chopped

    - 2 cups chopped fresh spinach

    - 1/2 cup Greek yogurt

- 1/4 cup grated Parmesan cheese

- 1/4 cup shredded mozzarella cheese

- 1/4 cup mayonnaise

- 1 clove garlic, minced

- Salt and pepper to taste

- Tortilla chips or vegetable sticks for dipping

- *Instructions:*

1. Preheat oven to 375°F (190°C).

2. In a bowl, mix together chopped artichoke hearts, chopped spinach, Greek yogurt, Parmesan cheese, mozzarella cheese, mayonnaise, minced garlic, salt, and pepper.

3. Transfer the mixture to a baking dish and smooth the top.

4. Bake for 25-30 minutes, or until the dip is bubbly and golden brown on top.

5. Serve hot with tortilla chips or vegetable sticks for dipping.

These recipes offer a variety of options for healthy, cancer-friendly snacks and desserts that are delicious and satisfying. Enjoy experimenting with different flavors and ingredients to find your favorites!

CONCLUSION

This cancer-friendly cookbook offers a comprehensive collection of nutritious and delicious recipes tailored to support individuals affected by cancer throughout their journey. From breakfast to dinner, snacks to smoothies, and everything in between, each recipe has been carefully crafted to provide nourishment, hydration, and comfort during treatment and recovery.

By focusing on cancer-friendly ingredients and cooking methods, this cookbook empowers readers to make health-conscious choices that promote overall well-being and support their body's needs during this challenging time. Whether managing treatment side effects, addressing nutritional deficiencies, or simply seeking flavorful and satisfying meals, the recipes presented here offer a variety of options to suit diverse tastes and preferences.

Beyond the kitchen, this cookbook also emphasizes the importance of hydration, mindful eating, and overall self-care as integral components of cancer management and survivorship. By incorporating hydrating beverages, nutrient-rich foods, and practical tips for meal planning and preparation, readers can take proactive steps to optimize their nutrition, manage treatment-related symptoms, and enhance their quality of life.

As individuals navigate the complex and often daunting landscape of cancer diagnosis and treatment, this cookbook serves as a valuable resource and source of inspiration, providing nourishment for both body and soul. With its wealth of cancer-friendly recipes, practical guidance, and words of encouragement, it is our hope that this cookbook will empower readers to embrace a healthy and flavorful approach to eating, fostering resilience, strength, and vitality on their journey toward wellness and healing.